Fast Facts:
Heart Failure

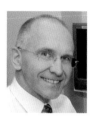

Dariusz Korczyk MD IntMedSpec(P)
FRACP FCSANZ MHFA
Cardiologist, Heart Failure Unit
Princess Alexandra Hospital
Brisbane, Australia

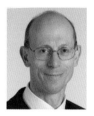

Thomas H Marwick MD PhD MPH
FRACP FESC FRCP FACC
Section Head, Cardiovascular Imaging
Heart and Vascular Institute, Cleveland Clinic
Professor of Medicine, Lerner College of Medicine
Case Western Reserve University, Cleveland, Ohio, USA

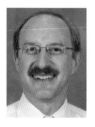

Gerry Kaye MBChB MD FRCP FRACP
Consultant Cardiologist and
Associate Professor of Cardiology
Department of Cardiology
Princess Alexandra Hospital
Brisbane, Australia

Declaration of Independence
This book is as balanced and as practical as we can make it.
Ideas for improvement are always welcome: feedback@fastfacts.com

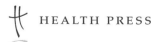

HEALTH PRESS

Fast Facts: Heart Failure
First edition August 2012

Text © 2012 Dariusz Korczyk, Thomas H Marwick, Gerry Kaye
© 2012 in this edition Health Press Limited

Health Press Limited, Elizabeth House, Queen Street, Abingdon,
Oxford OX14 3LN, UK
Tel: +44 (0)1235 523233
Fax: +44 (0)1235 523238

Book orders can be placed by telephone or via the website.
For regional distributors or to order via the website, please go to: fastfacts.com
For telephone orders, please call +44 (0)1752 202301 (UK, Europe and
Asia–Pacific), 1 800 247 6553 (USA, toll free) or +1 419 281 1802 (Americas).

Fast Facts is a trademark of Health Press Limited.

A CIP record for this title is available from the British Library.

ISBN 978-1-908541-28-4

Korczyk D (Dariusz)
Fast Facts: Heart Failure/
Dariusz Korczyk, Thomas H Marwick, Gerry Kaye

Medical illustrations by Dee McLean, London, and
Annamaria Dutto, Withernsea, UK.
Typesetting and page layout by Zed, Oxford, UK.
Printed by Latimer Trend & Company Limited, Plymouth, UK.

Text printed on biodegradable and recyclable paper
manufactured using elemental chlorine free (ECF) wood
pulp from well-managed forests.

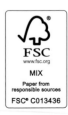

FSC
www.fsc.org
MIX
Paper from
responsible sources
FSC® C013436

Glossary and abbreviations

Afterload: the amount of hemodynamic pressure – peripheral vascular resistance – downstream from the heart

Amyloidosis: systemic illness with uncontrolled production and organ deposition of abnormal protein

BNP: type B natriuretic peptide

BP: blood pressure

Cachexia: loss of weight with muscle atrophy, fatigue, weakness and significant loss of appetite as a result of chronic illness

CAD: coronary artery disease

Compensated heart failure: heart failure with sufficient cardiac output maintained by physiological compensatory mechanisms

Contractile reserve: measure of the myocardium's ability to increase its contractility with stress (exercise or dobutamine)

Cor pulmonale: failure of the right side of the heart due to long-term high blood pressure in the pulmonary arteries and right ventricle.

CPAP: continuous positive airway pressure

CRT: cardiac resynchronization therapy (CRT-P, with pacemaker; CRT-D, with pacemaker and defibrillator)

CSA: central sleep apnea

Decompensated heart failure: heart failure with clinical signs of fluid overload or low-output state despite compensatory mechanisms

GFR: glomerular filtration rate

HFpEF: heart failure with preserved ejection fraction

Hypovolemia: intravascular volume loss (due to, for example, bleeding, dehydration, fluid loss)

ICD: implantable cardiac defibrillator

Inotropic: increasing the strength of myocardial contraction

Ischemic heart disease: cardiac disease resulting from CAD

Lusitropic: increasing myocardial relaxation

LV: left ventricle/ventricular

LVEF: left ventricular ejection fraction

LVH: left ventricular hypertrophy

MET: metabolic equivalent of task; defined as the ratio of metabolic rate during a specific physical activity to a reference metabolic rate. (MET values range from 0.9 [sleeping] to 18 [running at 17.5 km/hour])

MI: myocardial infarction

NYHA: New York Heart Association

Preload: passive filling of the heart

OSA: obstructive sleep apnea

RV: right ventricle/ventricular

TAH: total artificial heart

Vasoconstriction: active narrowing of the blood vessels (arteries) in response to a trigger

Introduction

Increasingly, heart failure (HF) is becoming a serious public health problem. Studies have shown that at the age of 40 the lifetime risk of developing HF is 1 in 5 (lifetime risk of developing cancer is 1 in 2–3). As life expectancy has increased, so has the number of patients requiring treatment and the associated cost to society. It is therefore imperative that every society implements strategies that deliver services to those in need and, more importantly, prevent the onset of the disease in at-risk individuals.

For centuries it was recognized that breathlessness and peripheral edema were related to an abnormality of cardiac function, while the dramatic effects of digoxin were demonstrated 250 years ago. However, it is only in the past 30 years or so that we have gained a better understanding of the mechanisms and outcomes of HF. As a result, effective new treatments, including pharmacotherapy, surgical interventions, transplantation and device therapy, have been developed, which have revolutionized both outcome and wellbeing in patients with HF. In fact, the area has changed so rapidly in recent years that management of HF has become an established specialty in its own right.

Fast Facts: Heart Failure succinctly explains recent therapeutic advances and their role in the modern management of HF. This book is an ideal introduction to HF for healthcare professionals working in primary care, cardiac nurses, junior hospital doctors, medical students and cardiology trainees. Our aim is to provide a concise overview of the mechanisms and the latest data on the underlying causes of HF, together with a clear approach to patient management – from drugs to surgery to devices – in a highly readable form.

Acknowledgments. The authors thank the following contributors from the Princess Alexandra Hospital, Brisbane, Australia: Drs RLC Adams and RJ Bird, for the section on anemia in Chapter 4 – Comorbidities; Mrs R Peters, nurse practitioner, for her contribution to Chapter 6 – General management and lifestyle considerations; and Mrs T Chang, pharmacist, for her contribution to Chapter 7 – Pharmacological treatment.

Definitions

The term 'heart failure' (HF) is generally used to describe the physiological state in which cardiac function is insufficient to meet the metabolic needs of the tissues. Detailed criteria for the diagnosis of HF (Framingham criteria and European Society of Cardiology guidelines) are given in Chapter 5 (see page 62). A complete description of the HF syndrome in every patient should also recognize the following entities:

- diastolic versus systolic
- acute versus chronic
- right versus left (and biventricular)
- high versus low output.

Each of these has implications for investigation, management and outcome.

Diastolic versus systolic heart failure. The outcome of these entities is similar, although their treatment is different. The definition of ejection fraction (the percentage of blood pumped from the ventricles with each heart beat) is fundamental to defining diastolic and systolic HF (Figure 1.1). An ejection fraction over 50% is generally regarded as normal, although there remains some debate regarding the specific cut-off point.

Systolic heart failure results from myocardial injury, which leads to impaired pumping function of the left ventricle (LV) and reduced LV ejection fraction (LVEF < 40%). This is the typical manifestation of patients with ischemic heart disease and multiple infarcts.

Diastolic heart failure. Normally, the driving force for diastolic filling is elastic recoil (suction) and relaxation of the LV due to the coordinated motion of myocardial fibers, which causes the twisting and untwisting of the heart. Diastolic HF is caused by abnormal LV suction (from untwisting), relaxation and chamber compliance, with resulting elevation in diastolic pressure. Diastolic HF is now more commonly known by the terms 'heart failure with preserved (or normal) ejection fraction' (HFpEF; HFnEF). It is the typical manifestation of patients with hypertensive heart disease and small ventricles with reduced stroke volume and filling

7

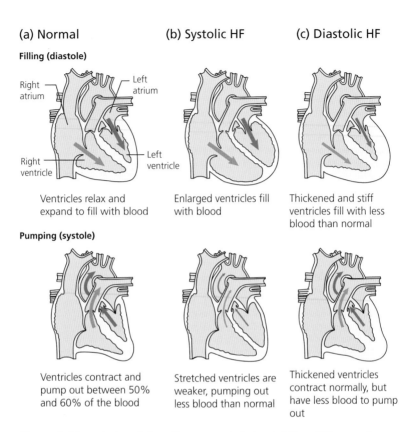

Figure 1.1 Description of diastolic versus systolic heart failure (HF), according to ejection fraction: (a) normal heart; (b) systolic HF; and (c) diastolic HF.

disturbances. HFpEF is common in the elderly (affecting more women than men) in whom combined ischemia, hypertrophy and age-related fibrosis may act together to produce increased myocardial stiffness and delayed relaxation. Prevalence increases with age.

Heart failure with normal systolic and diastolic function describes a group of patients with symptomatic HF but no evidence of systolic or diastolic dysfunction on resting echocardiography. In one study, 15% of patients with clinical HF had normal LVEF and normal tests of diastolic function at rest. Historically, these patients would have been diagnosed as having HFpEF, but dobutamine stress echocardiography has helped to reclassify about 60% of these patients with various diagnoses, including left ventricular outflow tract obstruction, development of restrictive filling pattern at stress, chronotropic incompetence or underlying ischemic heart disease.

In addition, some symptomatic patients do not have HF. Their symptoms may be caused by fluid overload (due to renal disease) or obesity and deconditioning.

Acute versus chronic heart failure. The terminology 'acute' and 'chronic' in this context relates to time rather than severity. An episode of acute HF can be defined as the sudden onset or gradual worsening of signs and symptoms of HF that results in hospital admission. The typical presentation of acute HF is pulmonary edema. Acute LV failure elevates LV diastolic pressure, which causes a significant rise in pulmonary venous pressure, resulting in pulmonary congestion (edema), as well as subendocardial ischemia, further LV remodeling and worsening of mitral valve regurgitation. The patient presents with severe dyspnea at rest, pink frothy sputum, sweating and clamminess, and sometimes shock. Raised right-sided filling pressure in response to LV dysfunction contributes to the development of systemic congestion with elevated jugular venous pressure and peripheral edema. The combination of poor cardiac output (in 50% of patients with acute HF) and renal venous hypertension may precipitate a worsening of renal function and could cause cardiorenal syndrome (see Chapter 4). In acute HF, the degree of pulmonary congestion (wet vs dry) and state of tissue perfusion (warm vs cold) varies (see Chapter 5).

HF that is provoked by an acute illness (e.g. myocardial infarction [MI]) may not be preceded by chronic symptoms. Conversely, chronic HF has a background of gradually worsening exertional dyspnea, edema, orthopnea and paroxysmal nocturnal dyspnea.

Recognizing the acuity of HF symptoms is an important aspect of managing HF as a chronic disease. Recognizing an exacerbation in a patient with chronic HF should lead to a search for the etiology of this change.

Right, left and biventricular failure. Left ventricular HF is the most common type of HF. It is associated with exertional dyspnea, orthopnea and paroxysmal nocturnal dyspnea. Right ventricular HF, most commonly caused by left ventricular HF, is characterized by edema, abdominal distension (due to ascites), right upper quadrant discomfort (due to liver congestion) and jugular venous pressure often with prominent v waves due to tricuspid regurgitation (see Chapter 5). Either left- or right-sided HF may occur in the context of low output (fatigue, syncope and hypotension).

High versus low output. The distinction between high- and low-output HF has etiologic and therapeutic implications. Low-output HF is associated with pale, cool extremities, which reflects vasoconstriction and reduced cardiac output. High-output HF is associated with warm extremities and bounding pulses. In its most extreme state, this entity is associated with HF due to arteriovenous shunts or diseases associated with severe vasodilation (e.g. vitamin B_1 deficiency – beri-beri).

Epidemiology

Over the past 40 years, advances in the treatment of acute coronary syndromes have reduced deaths from coronary artery disease (CAD), but the corollary has been an increase in the prevalence of newly diagnosed HF, the rates of first and recurrent HF hospitalizations and deaths from HF (Figure 1.2).

A growing problem. Recently, HF has emerged as a potential world health problem of epidemic proportions. Its enormous impact on individuals and

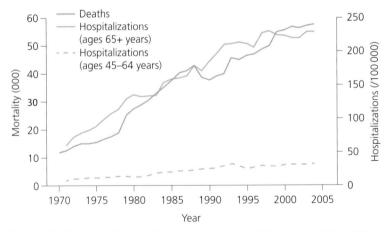

Figure 1.2 Deaths and hospitalizations due to heart failure in the USA, 1971–2004. The sharp drop in deaths in 1989 is attributed to the revision of the death certificate at that time. Adapted from Vital Statistics of the USA and National Hospital Discharge Survey, National Center for Health Statistics 2006.

their families is compounded by the huge costs to healthcare budgets around the world. The burden associated with HF is expected to rise over the next 20 years due to a number of factors:

- aging populations in developed countries
- increases in the number of elderly people with CAD and hypertension
- decreases in case–fatality rates associated with acute coronary syndromes
- improved diagnosis using sensitive techniques such as echocardiography.

The rising prevalence of obesity, metabolic syndrome and diabetes mellitus with associated cardiovascular complications is likely to result in further increases.

Some of the factors listed above cannot be modified (e.g. aging of the population), but prevention of those that precede the development of HF (CAD, diabetes mellitus, arterial hypertension) should be a priority.

Prevalence. An increase in the prevalence of HF in developed countries has been observed over time; current estimates are shown in Table 1.1. In those with CAD, a 28% decrease in 5-year mortality after MI was associated with a 25% increase in the 5-year rate of HF. About 70% of patients developed HF within 5 years, with two-thirds of clinical cases in the first year.

Incidence. The incidence of HF also increases with age. In the Framingham Heart Study, the incidence approximately doubled over each successive decade of life, rising more steeply with age in women than in men. The

---

TABLE 1.1

Prevalence of heart failure – current estimates

- 2–3% of the world's population is affected by symptomatic HF (~ 22 million people worldwide; 6.5 million in Europe; > 5 million in the USA; > 700 000 in the UK; > 350 000 in Australia)
- 8 per 1000 people aged 50–59 years are affected by HF*
- 66 per 1000 men aged 80–89 years are affected by HF*
- 79 per 1000 women aged 80–89 years are affected by HF*

*The known prevalence in African-Americans is around 25% higher.

annual incidence in men rises from 2 per 1000 at 35–64 years of age to 12 per 1000 at 65–94 years. The age-adjusted incidence has not, however, changed significantly over time.

While there are some geographic and demographic variations (reflecting differences in the most common etiologies of HF), approximately half of all incident cases of HF are either systolic or diastolic HF.

Hospitalization. The increase in prevalence has been associated with a three- to fourfold rise in the rate of hospitalization for HF. In 2004, there were over 1 million hospitalizations in the USA with a first-listed discharge diagnosis of HF. The rehospitalization rate following index admission with HF is high (about 50% at 6 months). However, approximately 50% of these readmissions are due to non-HF conditions (e.g. respiratory causes) and this rate is even higher in those over 65 years of age.

Acute heart failure. While a history of chronic HF can be established in 80% of patients, 20% present with de novo cardiac dysfunction. In 50% of admissions LV systolic function is normal or near normal (HFpEF). Most of this subgroup are elderly women of 75 years and older at presentation.

Mortality. Although comprehensive medical treatment, with attention to target drug doses (especially for beta-blockers), and the advent of device therapy have resulted in a significant drop in morbidity and mortality related to HF, mortality still exceeds that reported for most common malignancies (Figure 1.3).

HF has an annual mortality of 19%, with a median survival of 2.3 years in men and 1.7 years in women who require hospitalization for a first episode. However, as HF results from heterogeneous causes of cardiac damage, mortality rates vary. The worst outcomes have been reported with HF related to HIV infection, cardiac infiltration (amyloid) or cardiac cytotoxicity (due to anthracycline), while the mortality for CAD-related HF (ischemic cardiomyopathy) exceeds that of non-CAD-related HF. Conversely, HFpEF appears to have a better prognosis, with an annual mortality of 8–9% in some reports.

Predisposing conditions. CAD, arterial hypertension, valvular heart disease and diabetes mellitus are the four most important predisposing

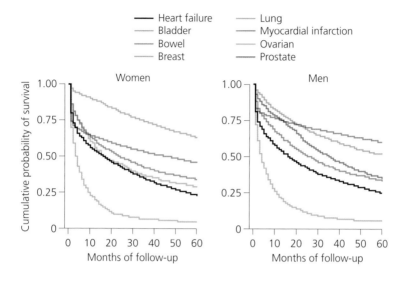

Figure 1.3 The prognosis of heart failure compared with that for common malignancies in men and women. Adapted from Stewart S et al. 2001.

conditions for the development of HF (see Chapter 3). Over the past 50 years, the prevalence of CAD and diabetes mellitus has increased, while rates of valvular heart disease and hypertension have fallen. Nevertheless, aortic valve disease and arterial hypertension remain the commonest causes of HFpEF in elderly people.

Population attributable risk estimates the proportion of HF in the population that is attributable to each predisposing condition. Available data suggest that for individuals over 65 years old CAD (13.1% annual risk), uncontrolled arterial hypertension (12.8%), C-reactive protein as a marker of vascular inflammation (9.7%) and low ankle–arm index (9.2%) have the largest effects, while low LVEF (4.1%) and atrial fibrillation (2.2%) have less effect than expected. Table 1.2 shows the relative risks and population attributable risks for some of the most common predisposing conditions.

Somewhat unexpected causes of HF have been found in patients in whom the initial diagnosis was not apparent: idiopathic (50%); myocarditis (9%);

ischemic heart disease (7%); infiltrative disease (5%); peripartum cardiomyopathy (4%); hypertension (4%); HIV infection (4%); connective tissue disease (3%); substance abuse (3%); and cytotoxicity (1%).

Additive risk. The presence of two or more predisposing conditions in the same individual increases the risk of developing HF. For example, in patients with hypertension an antecedent MI increases the risk by five to six times, while symptomatic CAD, diabetes mellitus, left ventricular hypertrophy and valve diseases each increase the risk by two to three times.

TABLE 1.2

Risk of heart failure from common predisposing conditions

	Relative risk	Overall 'population attributable risk' (%)
Coronary heart disease	8.1	62
Cigarette smoking	1.6	17
Hypertension	1.4	10
Overweight	1.3	8
Diabetes mellitus	1.9	3
Valvular heart disease	1.5	2

Key points – definitions and epidemiology

- Systolic heart failure (HF) is characterized by a reduction of ejection fraction to less than 40%.
- Symptomatic HF affects 2–3% of the global population.
- The financial burden associated with HF is likely to rise over the next 20 years.
- Overall prognosis is poor.
- Coronary artery disease, arterial hypertension, valvular heart disease and diabetes mellitus are the four most important predisposing conditions for the development of HF.

Key references

Bleumink GS, Knetsch AM, Sturkenboom MC et al. Quantifying the heart failure epidemic: prevalence, incidence rate, lifetime risk and prognosis of heart failure. The Rotterdam Study. *Eur Heart J* 2004;25:1614–19.

Bursi F, Weston SA, Redfield MM et al. Systolic and diastolic heart failure in the community. *JAMA* 2006;296: 2209–16.

Gottdiener JS, Arnold AM, Aurigemma GP et al. Predictors of congestive heart failure in the elderly: the Cardiovascular Health Study. *J Am Coll Cardiol* 2000;35:1628–37.

Havranek EP, Masoudi FA, Westfall KA et al. Spectrum of heart failure in older patients: results from the National Heart Failure project. *Am Heart J* 2002;143:412–17.

He J, Ogden LG, Bazzano LA et al. Risk factors for congestive heart failure in US men and women: NHANES I epidemiologic follow-up study. *Arch Intern Med* 2001;161:996–1002.

Jhund PS, Macintyre K, Simpson CR et al. Long-term trends in first hospitalization for heart failure and subsequent survival between 1986 and 2003: a population study of 5.1 million people. *Circulation* 2009;119:515–23.

Lloyd-Jones D, Adams RJ, Brown TM et al. Heart disease and stroke statistics – 2010 update: a report from the American Heart Association. *Circulation* 2010;121:e46–215.

Lloyd-Jones DM, Larson MG, Leip EP et al. Lifetime risk for developing congestive heart failure: the Framingham Heart Study. *Circulation* 2002;106:3068–72.

Mahadevan G, Davis RC, Frenneaux MP et al. Left ventricular ejection fraction: are the revised cut-off points for defining systolic dysfunction sufficiently evidence based? *Heart* 2008;94:426–8.

Masoudi FA, Havranek EP, Smith G et al. Gender, age, and heart failure with preserved left ventricular systolic function. *J Am Coll Cardiol* 2003;41:217–23.

McCullough PA, Philbin EF, Spertus JA et al. Confirmation of a heart failure epidemic: findings from the Resource Utilization Among Congestive Heart Failure (REACH) study. *J Am Coll Cardiol* 2002;39:60–9.

Stewart S, MacIntyre K, Hole DJ et al. More 'malignant' than cancer? Five-year survival following a first admission for heart failure. *Eur J Heart Fail* 2001;3:315–22.

Thomas MD, Fox KF, Wood DA et al. Echocardiographic features and brain natriuretic peptides in patients presenting with heart failure and preserved systolic function. *Heart* 2006;92:603–8.

Vasan RS, Larson MG, Benjamin EJ et al. Congestive heart failure in subjects with normal versus reduced left ventricular ejection fraction: prevalence and mortality in a population-based cohort. *J Am Coll Cardiol* 1999;33:1948–55.

Pathophysiology

Advances in the management of heart failure (HF) over the past 20 years have been informed by a better understanding of its pathophysiology. There are few situations in cardiology where treatment has been as closely linked to an appreciation of the underlying science.

Vicious cycle of heart failure. HF is a disease of inappropriate adaptation to injury. The body has a limited range of compensatory responses to circulatory impairment, mainly vasoconstriction and sodium and water retention (see below). In general, however, these adjustments to hypovolemia are poorly suited to pump failure, and increases in the preload and afterload of the failing heart lead to worsening HF (Figure 2.1).

Neurohormonal pathways. Sympathetic activation of the adrenergic system leads to vasoconstriction, which increases the resistance to blood flow and helps to maintain arterial pressure when cardiac output is reduced. However, vasoconstriction also increases afterload on the heart, leading to a worsening of HF (see Figure 2.1). Enhanced sympathetic outflow also activates the renin–angiotensin–aldosterone system

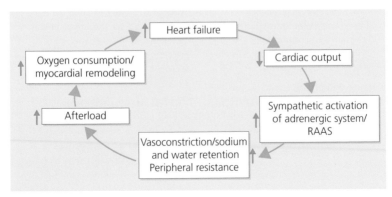

Figure 2.1 The vicious cycle of heart failure. RAAS, renin–angiotensin–aldosterone system.

(Figure 2.2). Renin release from the kidneys causes increased formation of angiotensin I from angiotensinogen and, via the action of angiotensin-converting enzyme (ACE), angiotensin II. Angiotensin II causes systemic vasoconstriction and acts on the adrenal cortex to produce aldosterone, leading to sodium and water retention. In addition, aldosterone (which may be released even in the setting of ACE inhibition) contributes to myocardial and vascular fibrosis. Sympathetic stimulation also releases antidiuretic hormone, which leads to retention of free water and contributes to dilutional hyponatremia.

Type B natriuretic peptide (BNP) is normally produced in response to atrial and ventricular distension and leads to increased sodium excretion and vasodilation, especially in the early phases of HF. In the end stage of HF the peptide may not be released because of myocyte loss.

Other pathways also reflect an inappropriate response to injury. Cytokine release is increased in HF, leading to a variety of consequences including apoptosis. The role of these as contributors to the progression of HF, rather than a correlate, is debated. Certainly, the failure of tumor necrosis factor (TNF) inhibitors to improve outcome argues against a causative role.

Remodeling of the myocardium. Global and local responses to maladaptive stimuli lead to myocardial remodeling, namely increased myocardial volume and mass and a net loss of myocytes. The heart has the ability to

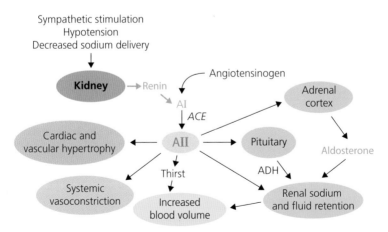

Figure 2.2 Neurohormonal pathways in heart failure. ACE, angiotensin-converting enzyme; ADH, antidiuretic hormone; AI/AII, angiotensin I/II.

change the force of contraction, and therefore stroke volume, in response to changes in venous return (the Frank–Starling mechanism). A reduction in stroke volume due to myocardial injury can be overcome by left ventricular (LV) enlargement. This is not a response that can keep occurring indefinitely – eventually a loss of LV function will occur due to reduced interaction between contractile elements, caused by their separation.

LV hypertrophy (LVH) maintains wall stress as the LV enlarges. However, it is also eventually maladaptive as the hypertrophied myocardium exceeds the growth of its blood supply.

Autonomic reflexes. The increase of sympathetic tone associated with HF leads to disturbance of the autonomic reflexes. Persistent elevation of the heart rate is maladaptive in the ventricle: disturbances of LV relaxation are common, so the shortening of diastole that occurs with tachycardia (the duration of systole remains stable) is not well tolerated.

Insulin resistance is an important metabolic sequel to HF. It contributes to the disturbance of myocyte energy metabolism, leading to the description of the failing heart as 'an engine out of fuel'. Causes of insulin resistance include the underlying etiologies of HF (central obesity, diabetes mellitus) and loss of skeletal muscle (see below).

Peripheral vasoconstriction, as described above, symptomatically may contribute to cold sensitivity.

Loss of skeletal muscle is an important manifestation of HF, reflecting inactivity, consequences of circulating substances such as tumor growth factor (TGF)-β and reduced cardiac output. In its most advanced manifestation, loss of skeletal muscle may lead to cachexia. The consequences of this process include contributions to insulin resistance as well as loss of the skeletal muscle circulatory bed. The loss of this vasculature represents an additional decrement in the amount of vasculature that can undergo vasodilation (and therefore unload the LV).

Cardiorenal interactions. Reduced renal perfusion in HF (due to reduced stroke volume and vasoconstriction) is an important contributor to sodium and fluid overload. The exact links between cardiac and renal function have yet to be resolved. More marked disturbances of renal function, leading to coexisting renal failure, may also occur and pose problems for volume control.

Clinical stages and functional classes

The clinical syndrome of HF represents the final manifestation of advanced disease. Although advances have been made in the management of this entity, the greatest hope of avoiding the adverse outcome of HF is to intervene at an earlier, subclinical stage, when there is more likelihood of reversing the process. In recognition of this, the American Cardiology Association (ACC)/American Heart Association (AHA) guidelines divide progression of the disease into four preclinical and clinical stages (Table 2.1).

TABLE 2.1

The clinical stages and functional classes of heart failure

ACC/AHA stage	Clinical status	NYHA class	Functional status
A	Preclinical: risk factors for HF but no structural heart disease or symptoms	I	No limitation in any activities; no symptoms from ordinary activities
B	Preclinical: structural evidence of heart disease, but no symptoms	I	No limitation in any activities; no symptoms from ordinary activities
C	Clinical: structural evidence of heart disease, and symptoms or signs of HF	I, II, III	No, slight (e.g. mild shortness of breath) or marked limitation of any activity due to symptoms; comfortable *only* at rest
D	Clinical: structural evidence of heart disease, and symptoms and signs of HF	II, III, IV	Slight or marked limitation of any activity; symptoms at rest

Adapted from the American College of Cardiology (ACC)/American Heart Association (AHA) 2001 guidelines and The Criteria Committee of the New York Heart Association (NYHA), *Nomenclature and Criteria for Diagnosis of Diseases of the Heart and Great Vessels*, 9th edn. Boston: Little, Brown & Co, 1994:253–6.

It is important to distinguish these from functional classes, as described in the New York Heart Association (NYHA) classification system, which is based on severity of symptoms and exercise capacity and can be used to assess response to treatment.

ACC/AHA stages A and B are preclinical; these patients fall into NYHA functional class I. ACC/AHA stage C reflects patients with symptoms or signs of HF, so these patients may be classified functionally in any of the NYHA classes I to III. The functional status of patients in ACC/AHA class D (with symptoms and signs of HF) is usually limited (NYHA class II to IV).

The association between functional class, cardiac function (LVEF) and prognosis is discussed in more detail in Chapter 9.

Key points – pathophysiology and clinical stages

- Heart failure (HF) is a disease of response to injury, which is initially appropriate and becomes inappropriate.
- Inappropriate non-cardiac responses include activation of a variety of hormonal reflexes (vasoconstriction, and sodium and water retention). Reversal of these inappropriate responses is critical to the management of HF.
- Remodeling is a cardiac response that is initially appropriate and becomes inappropriate as the heart enlarges excessively and hypertrophies.
- Symptoms develop in HF as a result of a complex web of interactions, involving not only the heart, hormonal changes and skeletal muscle, but also the vasculature (especially the endothelium), lungs and other organs.
- In addition to the classification of HF by clinical manifestation (acute versus chronic, systolic versus diastolic), etiology and precipitants (addressed in other chapters), HF can be classified by clinical stage (the course of the disease) and functional class (functional status based on symptom severity and exercise capacity).

Key references

National Heart Foundation of Australia. New York Heart Association (NYHA) grading of symptoms in congestive heart failure. In: *Guidelines for the Prevention, Detection and Management of Chronic Heart Failure in Australia*, 2011. Available at www.heartfoundation.org.au/ SiteCollectionDocuments/Chronic_ Heart_Failure_Guidelines_2011.pdf, last accessed 17 July 2012.

Piepoli MF, Guazzi M, Boriani G et al. Exercise intolerance in chronic heart failure: mechanisms and therapies. Part I. *Eur J Cardiovasc Prev Rehabil* 2010; 17:637–42.

Sica DA. Sodium and water retention in heart failure and diuretic therapy: basic mechanisms. *Cleve Clin J Med* 2006;73(Suppl 2):S2–7.

Triposkiadis F, Karayannis G, Giamouzis G et al. The sympathetic nervous system in heart failure physiology, pathophysiology, and clinical implications. *J Am Coll Cardiol* 2009;54:1747–62.

3 Causes

In the majority of patients with chronic heart failure (HF), clinical deterioration is caused by one factor or a combination of factors (Table 3.1). In de novo cases (acute HF), acute cardiac injury (either due to myocardial infarction [MI] or myocarditis) is the prevalent cause, although a sudden rise in afterload (uncontrolled blood pressure) or preload (intravenous fluid loading), extreme tachycardia or hypotension (as in acute anemia or sepsis) can result in cardiac compromise. Knowledge of the etiology is crucial in determining the optimal therapeutic strategy.

Ischemic heart disease
Ischemic heart disease is the commonest cause of left ventricular (LV) dysfunction and HF. It is characterized by a constant or intermittent decrease in coronary perfusion, caused by significant narrowing of the

TABLE 3.1

Causes of heart failure

Common	Rare
• Ischemic heart disease	• Thyroid disease
• Arterial hypertension	• Severe anemia
• Valvular heart disease	• Cardiotoxicity
• Primary cardiomyopathy	• Peripartum cardiomyopathy
• Diabetes mellitus	• Stress-provoked cardiomyopathy

Less common
- Infection and inflammation (myocarditis)
- Persistent arrhythmia
- Congenital heart disease
- Severe lung disease (cor pulmonale)
- Substance abuse (alcohol)

lumen of coronary arteries. This leads to a mismatch between the rate of oxygen delivery and the rate of its utilization by the cardiac muscle.

Coronary ischemia is usually due to coronary artery disease (CAD), in which an atherosclerotic lesion (plaque) develops within the wall of the coronary artery; when unstable, the plaque ruptures causing acute coronary occlusion and subsequent MI (Figure 3.1). Predisposing factors for the development of CAD are shown in Table 3.2.

Ischemic and non-ischemic cardiomyopathy. Ischemic cardiomyopathy is the term widely used to encompass coronary ischemia and MI with resulting myocardial scarring. In some patients, however, the degree of LV dysfunction is out of proportion to the magnitude of CAD. Such patients require further testing (invasive or non-invasive), as those with non-ischemic cardiomyopathy (i.e. not related to CAD) often present with typical angina, while those with CAD may have silent (asymptomatic) ischemia.

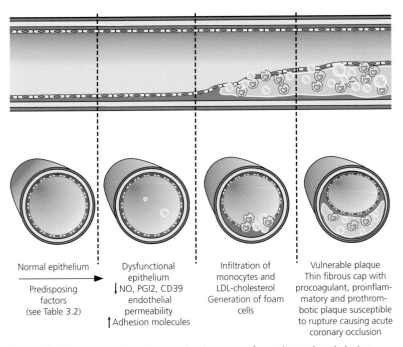

Normal epithelium	Dysfunctional epithelium	Infiltration of monocytes and	Vulnerable plaque Thin fibrous cap with
Predisposing factors (see Table 3.2)	↓NO, PGI2, CD39 endothelial permeability ↑Adhesion molecules	LDL-cholesterol Generation of foam cells	procoagulant, proinflammatory and prothrombotic plaque susceptible to rupture causing acute coronary occlusion

Figure 3.1 Coronary artery disease: development of an atherosclerotic lesion (plaque) in a coronary artery wall. CD39, cluster of differentiation 39; LDL, low-density lipoprotein; NO, nitric oxide; PGI2, prostaglandin I2 (prostacyclin).

TABLE 3.2

Predisposing factors for developing coronary artery disease

- Older age
- Male sex
- Family history
- Smoking

- Hyperlipidemia
- Arterial hypertension
- Diabetes mellitus
- Obesity

Over the past 25 years, mortality rates from acute coronary syndromes (MI and unstable angina) have declined, mainly as a result of improved and timely therapy to open the occluded artery (e.g. fibrinolysis, angioplasty, stenting). However, at the same time the rate of new presentation with HF has increased, indicating that many survivors of MI are left with or subsequently develop significant LV systolic dysfunction; some reports have indicated that more than 60% of individuals over 65 will develop HF within 2 years of MI.

The treatment of patients with non-ischemic cardiomyopathy (caused by infection, drugs, alcohol, arrhythmia etc.) and coexistent obstructive CAD is challenging, because the natural history of these patients is not predictable. The prognosis in many cases depends on the extent of CAD (number of vessels involved) and the presence of inducible coronary ischemia and myocardial scarring.

Arterial hypertension

Hypertension frequently develops between 35 and 60 years of age. In the developed world, arterial hypertension affects around 20% of the adult population. Although most have no identifiable cause (i.e. idiopathic hypertension), a family history of hypertension is common, so the proposed etiology includes interaction between polygenic mutations and environmental triggers. Secondary causes, which contribute to the development of hypertension in about 5% of cases, include primary adrenal disease (hyperaldosteronsim, hypercortisolemia, pheochromocytoma), hyperthyroidism, renal causes (including renal artery stenosis and parenchymal disease), sleep-disordered breathing, drugs, alcohol and others.

Hypertension and heart failure. Elevated arterial blood pressure (BP) is a common cause of LV hypertrophy (LVH) and may lead to LV diastolic and systolic dysfunction and overt HF. The development of LVH is associated with adverse outcomes and worse prognosis. The risk of developing HF increases with the degree of BP elevation; for example, a person with a BP of 160/100 mmHg or greater is twice as likely to develop HF as a person with a BP below 140/90 mmHg. Moderate elevations contribute to risk in the long term.

Pathological changes found in patients with LVH include an increase in the size of cardiac myocytes, progressive fibrosis, vascular changes of small arterioles with medial hypertrophy, and perivascular fibrosis.

The magnitude of LVH in response to a trigger such as hypertension depends not only on a direct response to the shear stress of raised pressure, but also the effect of changes in the levels of neurohormones, growth factors and cytokines. The reason why some hypertensive individuals progress directly to symptomatic LV systolic dysfunction without evidence of a significant cardiac event (MI) or diastolic HF is unknown.

Optimal BP control is an essential element of therapy in hypertensive heart disease. Evidence is emerging that tighter BP control (< 130/80 mmHg) is associated with reduction of LVH and cardiovascular events. Nonetheless, the role of tighter BP control remains controversial in the population as a whole and in certain subgroups, in particular diabetics and the elderly. Secondary causes of hypertension (including sleep-disordered breathing and renal artery stenosis) need to be ruled out in individuals with resistant hypertension and recurrent presentation with acute HF and elevated BP.

Valvular heart disease

Aortic valve stenosis. The most common cause of aortic valve stenosis is age-related valve degeneration, a result of ongoing inflammation with lipid deposition and progressive calcification. Congenital bicuspid aortic valve stenosis may be found in middle-aged populations. Rheumatic fever remains an important cause of aortic valve stenosis in areas of lower socioeconomic status.

Progressive aortic stenosis leads to exertional symptoms, such as dyspnea, chest pain and syncope, and the development of congestive HF. The emergence of symptoms heralds a worse prognosis (50% survival for 2–3 years) and dictates the need for aortic valve replacement. Historically, poor surgical candidates were managed medically or palliated with balloon valvuloplasty. However, the emergence of transcatheter aortic valve implantation (TAVI) with acceptable initial results provides an alternative for patients for whom corrective surgery is not appropriate.

Aortic valve stenosis and left ventricular dysfunction. Patients with severe aortic valve stenosis and LV systolic dysfunction (ejection fraction < 40%) are a challenging group to manage. They often present with a relatively low pressure gradient on echocardiography but with severe symptoms of HF. Importantly, the cause of HF (i.e. primary valvular disease versus primary myopathic process) has to be determined first, as the therapeutic options are different (surgery versus medical treatment). Patients without appropriate contractile reserve (on stress echocardiography) generally have a poor prognosis with either medical or surgical management, but may still benefit from aortic valve replacement.

Aortic valve regurgitation can be acute or chronic. Acute regurgitation, which presents with acute dyspnea and HF, is a cardiac emergency. Causes include perforation of aortic cusps in the course of bacterial endocarditis, proximal extension of a dissecting aortic aneurysm, trauma or dehiscence of an aortic prosthesis. Chronic regurgitation results from congenital, infective (syphilis), rheumatic or degenerative causes. Symptoms include progressive dyspnea, angina and symptoms of HF. Symptomatic patients have a much higher mortality rate than asymptomatic patients, and the severity of preoperative symptoms is a strong determinant of survival after valve replacement.

Mitral valve regurgitation is one of the commonest valvular diseases leading to HF. It poses a major diagnostic and therapeutic dilemma, as the distinction between organic (primary) and functional (secondary) causes, and thus the need for surgery, is not always obvious (Table 3.3).

Acute regurgitation – rupture of the papillary muscle or chordae tendineae due to endocarditis, cardiac ischemia or trauma – is a cardiac emergency. It manifests with severe dyspnea at rest, chest pain and symptoms of pulmonary edema. Chronic regurgitation leads to progressive breathlessness, initially on effort, with the development of symptoms of HF. Atrial arrhythmias are common. Symptomatic patients with severe primary mitral regurgitation are treated with surgery (valve repair or replacement).

TABLE 3.3

Causes of mitral valve regurgitation

Primary (organic)	Secondary (functional)
• Rheumatic heart disease	• Apical displacement of the papillary muscles (due to global LV remodeling)
• Valve prolapse	
• Valvular degenerative disease	• Dilation of mitral annulus (in dilated cardiomyopathy)
• Chordal rupture due to endocarditis, trauma or myocardial infarction	• Inferior LV wall remodeling (after infarction with displacement of the posterior papillary muscle)

Secondary mitral valve regurgitation (in patients with cardiomyopathy and CAD) is primarily a disease of the LV myocardium. Therapies that promote the reversal of LV remodeling, such as myocardial revascularization, beta-blocker therapy and cardiac resynchronization, should be instituted first. New percutaneous techniques for poor surgical candidates have emerged but require long-term data. Surgery should be considered in selected cases.

Mitral valve stenosis. The prevalence of mitral valve stenosis has declined in developed countries due to early recognition and treatment of rheumatic fever (its main cause). However, the resurgence of the disease has been observed in areas of lower socioeconomic status. Mitral valve stenosis causes progressive dyspnea and palpitations. Untreated, it leads to severe pulmonary hypertension and may result in right-sided HF characterized by peripheral edema and abdominal distension. Percutaneous (valvuloplasty) or surgical (valve replacement) treatment is required.

Tricuspid valve regurgitation often accompanies advanced left-sided heart or pulmonary disease, due to annular dilatation and non-closure of the valve leaflets. Rare causes of structural tricuspid valve regurgitation include endocarditis, rheumatic heart disease and trauma. Isolated severe tricuspid valve regurgitation may lead to right ventricular dysfunction and symptoms of right-sided HF. Symptoms of left-sided heart or pulmonary disease are prominent in most secondary cases.

Pulmonary valve stenosis is usually congenital, either isolated or part of a more complex congenital heart disease (e.g. tetralogy of Fallot). Symptoms include dyspnea and progressive right-sided HF.

Pulmonary valve regurgitation often occurs after surgical repair of a narrowed right ventricular outflow tract (with or without native valve excision) in patients with congenital heart disease (e.g. tetralogy of Fallot). Isolated significant pulmonary valve regurgitation is rare and caused by either endocarditis or hepatic carcinoid. Symptoms include right-sided HF and arrhythmia.

Patient prosthesis mismatch. All prosthetic valves are, to some degree, stenotic. Underestimating the size of the prosthesis at the time of aortic valve replacement may lead to persistence of LV hypertrophy and retard negative LV remodeling. Patient prosthesis mismatch during aortic valve replacement contributes to increased cardiac mortality rates, especially in patients with depressed LV function.

Cardiomyopathies

Cardiomyopathies are cardiac diseases in which the myocardium is a primary target of the pathological processes, characterized by abnormal chamber size and wall thickness or functional contractile dysfunctions. In 'primary cardiomyopathies' the cause is myocardial specific, whereas 'secondary cardiomyopathies' have a pre-existing cardiac (valvular disease, coronary ischemia, congenital heart disease or arrhythmia) or systemic (arterial hypertension, infective, hormonal or metabolic) cause.

The American Heart Association's proposed classification of cardiomyopathies is based on the etiology – genetic, acquired or mixed (Table 3.4) – rather than the cardiac phenotype. However, terms based on phenotype (dilated, restrictive and hypertrophic) remain in common use.

Genetic cardiomyopathies

Hypertrophic cardiomyopathy is an autosomal dominant genetic disorder of the heart muscle, in which a multitude of mutated genes encode compromised proteins of the cardiac sarcomere. At least 11 abnormal sarcomeric genes are implicated, which may partly explain the wide clinical presentation of the disease. Family members should be screened.

TABLE 3.4

Classification of primary cardiomyopathies

Genetic	Mixed	Acquired
• Hypertrophic	• Dilated	• Inflammatory (myocarditis)
• Arrhythmogenic right ventricular cardiomyopathy/ dysplasia	• Restrictive (non-hypertrophied and non-dilated)	• Stress-provoked (tako-tsubo)
• Isolated left ventricular non-compaction		• Peripartum
		• Tachycardia-induced
• Glycogen-storage diseases		• Infants of insulin-dependent diabetic mothers
– Danon disease		
– Pompe disease		
• Conduction defects		
• Mitochondrial myopathies		
• Ion channel disorders		
– Long QT syndrome		
– Brugada syndrome		
– Short QT syndrome		
– CPVT		
– Asian SUNDS		

CPVT, catecholaminergic polymorphic ventricular tachycardia; SUNDS, sudden unexpected nocturnal death syndrome.
Adapted from Maron BJ et al. 2006. American Heart Association Scientific Statement.

The disorder is characterized by an abnormal thickening of the left ventricle (Figure 3.2), usually in the absence of other conditions that increase ventricular pressure loading (e.g. systemic hypertension, aortic valve disease, the athlete's heart). All patients with hypertrophic cardiomyopathy require cardiologic referral, and syncope requires urgent investigation. The reported prevalence in the general population is about 0.2% (1:500), although true prevalence may be higher as it is often asymptomatic initially.

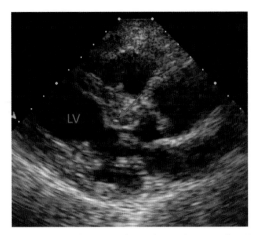

Figure 3.2 Hypertrophic cardiomyopathy: echocardiogram showing abnormal thickening of the septum (arrow). LV, left ventricle.

The disease has acquired a number of different names: asymmetric septal hypertrophy, idiopathic hypertrophic subaortic stenosis, muscular subaortic stenosis and hypertrophic obstructive cardiomyopathy. Although common, LV outflow obstruction is not a consistent feature and the term hypertrophic cardiomyopathy is now generally accepted as the name for this condition. In pregnancy, there is no convincing evidence that hypertrophic cardiomyopathy increases risk, but all patients should be offered obstetric and cardiologic care at specialized centers experienced in treating such conditions. Normal delivery is possible, but patients with severe outflow obstruction require special care and possibly Cesarean section.

Arrhythmogenic right ventricular cardiomyopathy/dysplasia is an uncommon genetic condition characterized by fibrofatty infiltration of the right ventricle. Both autosomal dominant and recessive inheritance have been described and a number of genes have been implicated. It is an important cause of sudden cardiac death, particularly in the young and usually due to a ventricular arrhythmia, or patients may manifest signs of right-sided HF and eventually biventricular failure.

Isolated left ventricular non-compaction is an idiopathic form of cardiomyopathy due to intrauterine arrest of myocardial compaction.

It was originally described in infants but more recently reported in adults. Both sporadic and familial forms are recognized. There is a spectrum of clinical presentation, and recent clinical reports have suggested that the disorder is associated with the important complications of thromboembolism, congestive HF, ventricular arrhythmias and sudden cardiac death.

Glycogen-storage diseases are rare genetic causes of cardiomyopathy. They include Danon disease (also known as lysosomal glycogen-storage disease with normal acid maltase) and Pompe disease (an autosomal recessive disorder characterized by the deficiency of acid alpha-glucosidase, a lysosomal hydrolase).

Mixed cardiomyopathies

Dilated cardiomyopathy is characterized by an increase in LV end-diastolic diameter (> 2.7 cm/m^2) (Figure 3.3) and reduced LV systolic function (ejection fraction < 45%). Most cases of dilated cardiomyopathy are idiopathic, but 35–50% of cases have a family history, usually suggesting an autosomal dominant inheritance.

In addition, about 10% of asymptomatic relatives have evidence of unrecognized LV dysfunction. Familial dilated cardiomyopathy (FDCM) can be further divided into two subtypes – isolated FDCM and FDCM with cardiac conduction defects. The latter subtype typically presents in

(a)   (b)

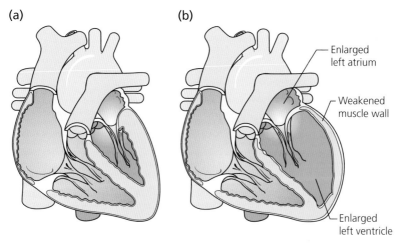

Enlarged
left atrium

Weakened
muscle wall

Enlarged
left ventricle

Figure 3.3 (a) Normal heart; and (b) dilated cardiomyopathy.

31

the second decade with mild cardiac conduction defects, which often progress to complete heart block. The responsible mutation was identified in the lamin A/C gene.

Restrictive cardiomyopathies are heterogeneous myocardial diseases with a common clinical picture of progressive symptoms of HF, including dyspnea, fatigue and exercise intolerance and varying degrees of peripheral edema, due to abnormal (restrictive) diastolic filling which results in a marked increase in ventricular end-diastolic pressures. Systolic function is usually preserved at least until the very advanced stage of the disease. A normal LV thickness differentiates this group from hypertrophic cardiomyopathies (see Figure 3.2); however, advanced stages of some of the diseases (e.g. cardiac amyloid) may present with marked LV hypertrophy.

Restrictive cardiomyopathies are caused by inflammatory, infiltrative or storage diseases (Figure 3.4), or are idiopathic. Some forms are triggered by mutations in the genes responsible for synthesis of the sarcomeric proteins, similar to those already identified in hypertrophic cardiomyopathy (see above).

The prognosis is poor, with death or heart transplantation usually within the first few years after diagnosis. The treatment to control HF is particularly difficult because of diuretic-resistant edema, medication

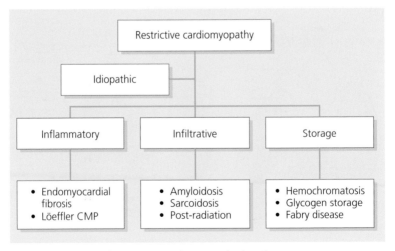

Figure 3.4 Causes of restrictive cardiomyopathy (CMP).

intolerance and drug toxicity leading to hypotension and arrhythmias. Underlying conduction disease also limits treatment choices and requires pacing in some cases.

Cardiac amyloidosis. The heart is one of the many organs involved in systemic amyloidosis. Secondary amyloidosis is seldom associated with important cardiac involvement. Primary amyloidosis typically presents with progressive deposition of abnormal protein (monoclonal immunoglobulin light chain) in multiple tissues and organs including the heart, kidneys, nervous system, skin and liver. Less than 5% have disease limited to the heart, while 20% of cases are caused by hematologic disorders (lymphoma, myeloma or macroglobulinemia).

Senile systemic amyloidosis is a slow progressive cardiomyopathy found mainly in patients over 80 years of age. It is caused by deposition of amyloid fibrils from plasma protein called transthyretin. The disease occurs more often in males and may present with isolated cardiac involvement and carpal tunnel syndrome.

Hereditary systemic amyloidosis with prominent cardiac involvement is caused by a mutation in the transthyretin gene, and is frequently found in African-Americans.

Management of cardiac amyloidosis includes supportive therapy for HF and arrhythmia, treatment of underlying amyloid disease and, in isolated cases, cardiac transplantation, although this is rarely an option because of the involvement of other organs and deposition of amyloid in the donor heart. Recently, combined heart and stem cell transplantation in young adults with preserved kidney, liver and autonomic function has shown promising results.

Fabry disease is an X-linked recessive lysosomal storage disorder caused by the absence of alpha-galactosidase A activity and the resultant accumulation of globotriaosylceramide and related glycosphingolipids. Severe forms of the disease (the classic phenotype) have no or just detectable residual enzyme activity, while variant forms have low enzyme levels. Typically, males are affected, but female carriers may have varying forms of cardiac and cerebrovascular disease due to random X-chromosome inactivation.

The disease is progressive in nature and the classic form has its onset in childhood. The symptoms are initially subtle or non-specific. By adulthood, specific organ involvement is fully established. Affected individuals present with renal failure requiring dialysis, cerebrovascular disease with transient ischemic attacks, strokes and complications of vascular disease, cutaneous angiokeratomas and characteristic corneal opacities. Cardiac involvement includes LV hypertrophy, valvular disease with predominant mitral insufficiency, ascending aortic aneurysm formation, CAD and conduction disease. Patients may present with symptoms of HF, arrhythmia or MI. Specific enzyme-replacement therapy (ERT) should be started early, ideally before end-organ damage. Treatment otherwise remains supportive.

Cardiac sarcoid. Sarcoidosis is a systemic disease with chronic inflammation and non-caseating granulomas in affected organs. Women are at slightly higher risk, with rates peaking at 20 to 29 years of age. Extracardiac manifestations occur in the skin (erythema nodosum), eyes (uveitis), lungs (interstitial infiltrates and adenopathy), kidneys (nephrocalcinosis, progressive renal failure) and parotid gland (swelling), and there may be hypocalcemia (abnormal calcium absorption).

Conduction disease is the commonest cardiac presentation; complete heart block is not uncommon. Ventricular arrhythmia is seen in up to a quarter of patients, atrial tachyarrhythmia less frequently.

Diagnosis requires a finding of granulomatous inflammation with giant cell formation on endomyocardial biopsy in patients with suspicious cardiac abnormalities (Figure 3.5). The serum level of angiotensin-converting enzyme (ACE) is not specific and results may be affected by inhibitors.

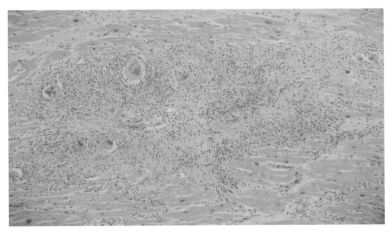

34   **Figure 3.5** Granulomatous myocarditis with giant cell formation.

Treatment of cardiac sarcoid includes disease-specific therapy with oral steroids (and immunosuppressive drugs) and supportive therapy, with HF medications, pacing and an implanted defibrillator in advanced conduction disease and life-threatening arrhythmia.

Hemochromatosis is an autosomal recessive disorder in which the *HFE* gene mutation C282Y (chromosome 6) reduces the affinity of transferrin for its receptor, resulting in the accumulation of iron in multiple organs including the liver, heart, pancreas, pituitary, joints and skin. C282Y homozygotes account for most clinical diagnoses of hereditary hemochromatosis among people of northern European descent.

Iron deposition may lead to restricted or dilated cardiomyopathies. Conduction disease including sinus node disease may coexist. In up to 15% of cases cardiac involvement may precede the involvement of other organs. The therapy of the condition includes iron removal (phlebotomy) as soon as the diagnosis is made. Established cardiac disease is rarely responsive to therapy.

Endomyocardial fibrosis is an idiopathic disorder characterized by the development of restrictive cardiomyopathy. It is sometimes considered part of a spectrum of a single disease process that includes Löeffler endocarditis (non-tropical eosinophilic endomyocardial fibrosis or fibroblastic parietal endocarditis with eosinophilia). It can cause progressive HF, thromboembolism, myocardial ischemia, arrhythmias and, rarely, pericarditis. Prognosis is poor. Therapy includes management of the underlying cause, the treatment of HF, arrhythmia and thromboembolism, and heart transplantation in selected cases.

Acquired cardiomyopathies

Inflammatory cardiomyopathy. The presentation of acute myocarditis may include general systemic symptoms (fever and malaise) associated with cardiac-specific complaints, including chest pain, symptoms of HF, palpitations and syncope. Clinical signs of cardiomyopathy may be florid and may be associated with arrhythmia (atrial and ventricular) and the potential for sudden cardiac death.

Acute myocarditis predominantly has an infective etiology (mainly viral) and many patients will recover their cardiac function. The more aggressive forms of myocarditis (giant cell [Figure 3.6] and eosinophilic necrotizing myocarditis) have characteristics of autoimmune disease and

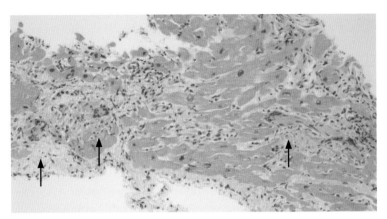

Figure 3.6 Giant cell myocarditis, i.e. myocytolysis with formation of giant cells (arrows). Biopsy in such cases is diagnostic.

poor prognosis. Chronic viral cardiomyopathy has been identified as a separate entity but the role of antiviral therapy in this condition has not yet been proved.

Stress-provoked (tako-tsubo) cardiomyopathy is an increasingly recognized cause of reversible LV cardiomyopathy, which occurs in around 2% of acute coronary syndromes. It occurs more often in women, usually after menopause, typically in circumstances of acute and severe emotional stress, hence it has been referred to as the 'broken heart syndrome'. Tako-tsubo cardiomyopathy is characterized by typical ischemic chest pain, ST segment elevation and an increase in cardiac enzymes, mimicking a full-thickness MI. Often, the coronary arteries show little or no disease. The left ventricle shows a characteristic abnormality on echocardiography and sometimes on angiography, that of apical hypo- or akinesis (otherwise it looks like a true infarct) and significant dilatation (ballooning) (Figure 3.7). Due to the way it presents, treatment is usually the same as that for an infarct: beta-blockers, ACE inhibitors, statins and an antiplatelet agent. Although it can present dramatically with cardiogenic shock or HF, with supportive treatment in-hospital mortality is usually low. The overall long-term prognosis is excellent.

Peripartum cardiomyopathy (PCM) is rare in developed countries and in white populations, but is ten times more common in African and African-

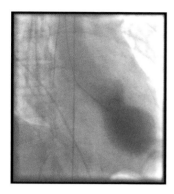

Figure 3.7 Left ventriculography during systole in a patient with tako-tsubo cardiomyopathy, showing ballooning of the apex, usually associated with apical hypo- or akinesis.

American women (e.g. affecting 1 in 300 live births in Haiti). The diagnostic criteria of PCM include:

- HF presenting in the last month of pregnancy and 5 months after delivery
- lack of other causes of cardiomyopathy
- no pre-existing heart disease before pregnancy.
  Risk factors are shown in Table 3.5.

PCM has an uncertain etiology associated with pregnancy. It is potentially fatal if not recognized and treated early. Recent work has focused on the beneficial effects of prolactin inhibition with bromocriptine. In general, however, the prognosis is good and relapses are uncommon.

Tachycardia-induced cardiomyopathy. A long-standing, persistently raised ventricular rate due to a supraventricular rhythm is a well-recognized cause of non-ischemic cardiomyopathy and HF. Its recognition is important as treatment often reverses HF and LV damage.

TABLE 3.5

Risk factors for peripartum cardiomyopathy

• Multiparity	• Pre-eclampsia
• Advanced age (> 30 years)	• Gestational hypertension
• Twin pregnancies	• African origin

Patients may present with exertional dyspnea, orthopnea and peripheral edema, but initially it is often difficult to determine whether the arrhythmia caused the HF or vice versa. The diagnosis can usually be inferred if LV function improves after successful treatment of the arrhythmia.

The most common tachycardias are atrial fibrillation and flutter; less commonly, atrial tachycardia and re-entrant atrial arrhythmias. Rarely, persistent ventricular tachycardia may present as HF. Paroxysmal tachycardias are rarely implicated as a cause of non-ischemic cardiomyopathy.

The common link is a persistently elevated ventricular rate, often more than 100 beats per minute, sometimes over a long period of time, even years. However, the heart rate itself is not a good predictor of HF. Although there is experimental evidence showing that the faster the heart rate the more likely LV impairment becomes, it is usually the slower but incessant arrhythmias that are associated with non-ischemic cardiomyopathy in humans.

Tachycardia-induced cardiomyopathy can occur at any age but it is rare in childhood. Atrial fibrillation and flutter are common in older age groups. The aim of treatment is to control the ventricular rate (either through rhythm or rate control), which should alleviate symptoms of HF, improve LV function and prevent future relapses (see *Fast Facts: Cardiac Arrhythmias*).

Athlete's heart. Long-term physical training, particularly in competitive athletes, can lead to a physiological increase in LV mass. To differentiate between athlete's heart and hypertrophic cardiomyopathy (see pages 28–30), training should be stopped for 4–6 weeks to demonstrate regression of the LV thickening. If hypertrophic cardiomyopathy is diagnosed, and particularly if there is an outflow gradient, the patient should be advised to stop taking part in extreme or competitive sports.

Diabetes mellitus and metabolic cardiomyopathies

HF has been called the 'forgotten complication' of diabetes mellitus. Indeed, this association appears to be bidirectional, as diabetes is associated with HF, and HF with impaired glucose tolerance and diabetes. Moreover, the development of HF is associated with worse outcome in diabetic compared to non-diabetic subjects, particularly in those with ischemic heart disease. This observation has led to the hypothesis that the diabetic heart is in some way compromised to the extent that it is less able to sustain injury from an exogenous insult such as MI.

Indeed, sophisticated imaging techniques have demonstrated a reduction of diastolic and systolic function in apparently healthy subjects with type 2 diabetes mellitus. This is a frequent observation, with various manifestations reported in 20% to more than 50% of apparently healthy diabetic subjects. These findings are also present in patients who have similar metabolic diseases, including impaired glucose tolerance and obesity, and a unifying feature may be insulin resistance. This subclinical dysfunction is multifactorial, with contributions from disturbed metabolism, fibrosis, microvascular disease (both structural and functional) and diabetic autonomic neuropathy. It is further magnified by the presence of hypertension, and occurs most commonly in individuals with poor glycemic control.

As these findings have been detected using highly sensitive new techniques, there has been some concern that they represent an echocardiographic curiosity rather than a disease. However, follow-up studies have shown an association with the subsequent development of HF.

Given the increasing frequency of both obesity and type 2 diabetes mellitus, the subclinical cardiomyopathy associated with these conditions may prove to be extremely important. At present, no clear treatment has been described, although there is evidence that dysfunction is reduced with improved glycemic control, weight reduction and exercise training (see *Fast Facts: Diabetes Mellitus*). The extent to which fibrosis may contribute to uncomplicated diabetes mellitus remains controversial. Inhibitors of the renin–angiotensin–aldosterone system have shown some promise, but a persuasive outcome trial is still awaited.

Cardiotoxicity

Cardiotoxicity is one of the most serious side effects of cancer therapy (chemotherapy, and mediastinal and neck radiation). It may manifest as cardiomyopathy, pericarditis, congestive HF, valvular heart disease or premature CAD.

Anthracycline chemotherapy (e.g. doxorubicin) is by far the most common cause of cardiomyopathy in cancer survivors. Acute toxicity is unlikely with current regimens. Chronic toxicity (development of cardiomyopathy within 1 year of therapy) and late onset (development of cardiomyopathy from years to decades after therapy) are all dose dependent. Other agents that have been associated with cardiotoxicity include cyclophosphamide, ifosfamide, cisplatin, carmustine, busulfan, mechlorethamine and mitomycin.

Cardiac events have also been reported with paclitaxel, etoposide, teniposide, the vinca alkaloids, 5-fluorouracil, cytarabine, amsacrine, cladarabine, asparaginase, tretinoin and pentostatin. However, an association with late cardiotoxicity has not been established for these agents.

Recent advances in cancer diagnosis have led to the discovery of mutations or amplifications in the kinases in malignant cell lineages. Therapy with tyrosine kinase inhibitors (e.g. trastuzumab, imatinib) devised to target these molecules has so far been very successful, leading to the expansion of indications and a proliferation of new agents. The targeted proteins are regulatory enzymes responsible for cell division, growth and apoptosis, so it is not surprising that cardiac toxicities have been encountered.

Cardiac surveillance of cancer therapy should include an annual history and physical examination. A baseline echocardiogram should be performed, with subsequent frequency based on age of treatment, cumulative dose and concomitant chest irradiation (for an anthracycline-based regimen). In established cases the drug should be stopped and therapy reviewed. An ACE inhibitor could be considered for subclinical LV dysfunction, with HF treatment introduced if the patient becomes symptomatic.

Common causes of worsened heart failure

There are a number of cardiac and non-cardiac factors not directly related to the biology of HF that may worsen the symptoms of HF and lead to acute hospitalization (Table 3.6). Identification, prevention and early treatment of these form the target for disease management programs.

TABLE 3.6

Common causes of worsened heart failure

Cause and effect	Action
Dietary indiscretion	
• Excessive sodium and water intake are well-recognized precipitating factors for readmission	• Restrict salt intake to < 2 g/day • Limit fluid intake to 1.5–2.0 L/day
Fluid excess	
• Excessive administration of intravenous fluids may worsen HF in certain clinical conditions (e.g. sepsis, after surgery)	• Careful monitoring of volume status
Medication non-adherence	
• Loss of therapeutic effect	• Address the reasons for non-adherence (e.g. patient fear of side effects, financial constraints or service access issues)
Uncontrolled arterial hypertension (BP > 140/90 mmHg)	
• An important precipitant of HF	• Antihypertensive therapy
• Particularly frequent in elderly patients with LVH and diastolic dysfunction	• Search for secondary causes, e.g. excessive salt or liquorice intake, drugs (NSAIDs) or renal artery stenosis
Progressive cardiac dysfunction	
• Ongoing cardiac remodeling	• Step up HF therapy and optimize current therapy • Introduce new agents • Consider ancillary therapy (pacemakers) or mechanical cardiac support • Check for the presence of associated non-cardiac precipitants (e.g. infection, metabolic derangement, toxins, drugs)

(CONTINUED)

TABLE 3.6 (CONTINUED)

Cause and effect	Action
Atrial arrhythmias	
• Loss of atrial contraction contributes to decreased LV filling and cardiac output • Uncontrolled atrial rhythm with fast ventricular response further limits diastolic time and worsens hemodynamics • Sudden deterioration may be accompanied by symptoms of coronary ischemia and low BP	• Treat the arrhythmia (see *Fast Facts: Cardiac Arrhythmias*)
Myocardial ischemia/infarction	
• Acute coronary ischemia is a common precipitant of HF deterioration	• Immediate medical therapy to stabilize the ruptured plaque (heparins, antiplatelet agents, statins) • Careful evaluation for percutaneous or surgical revascularization • Coronary angiography and intervention for patients with HF complicating acute coronary syndromes, and for patients with angina and non-ischemic cardiomyopathy
Acute or progressive renal dysfunction	
• Indicates progression of cardiac dysfunction and low output • Leads to sodium and water retention and progressive volume overload • Coexisting factors may worsen HF (rise in BP, poor metabolism of drugs leading to cardiotoxicity or progressive anemia)	• See Chapter 4, Cardiorenal syndrome

(CONTINUED)

TABLE 3.6 (CONTINUED)

Cause and effect	Action
Cardiac pacing	
• Patients with indications for permanent pacing (advanced AV block) may develop progressive HF symptoms • Pacemaker-dependent patients (with prolonged RV pacing) fare worst	• Implantation of LV lead
Pulmonary disease	
• Patients with COPD are more susceptible to pulmonary infection and worsening HF	• See Chapter 4, Pulmonary disease
Anemia	
• Impairs oxygen delivery to tissues and if abrupt (in cases of bleeding) may lead to organ hypoperfusion and sympathetic activation	• See Chapter 4, Anemia
Thyroid disease	
• Both hypo- and hyperthyroidism exacerbate HF	• Evaluate thyroid function in all acute presentations
Medications	
• The following drugs can precipitate worsening HF: antiarrhythmics (flecainide, sotalol), non-dihydropiridine calcium-channel blockers, glitazones, NSAIDs, COX-2 inhibitors, TCAs, theophylline, beta-agonist bronchodilators, OTC drugs with pseudoephedrine, corticosteroids, chemotherapeutics (anthracycline, taxanes etc.)	• Evaluate and monitor the patient's cardiac and non-cardiac drug regimen

AV, atrioventricular; BP, blood pressure; COPD, chronic obstructive pulmonary disease; COX-2 cyclooxygenase-2; HF, heart failure; LV, left ventricle; LVH, left ventricular hypertrophy; NSAID, non-steroidal anti-inflammatory drug; OTC, over the counter; RV, right ventricular; TCA, tricyclic antidepressant.

Key points – causes

- Ischemic heart disease is the commonest cause of left ventricular dysfunction and heart failure (HF).
- Arterial hypertension is an important cause of new presentation but also a powerful precipitant of acute worsening of existing HF.
- Aortic valve disease is an important cause of HF. Surgery is the best therapy for whom it is appropriate; assessment of severity in the context of existing cardiac dysfunction can be challenging, but helps to define individuals who would benefit most from surgery.
- Surgery is always required for organic mitral valve regurgitation, but if the cause is functional then surgery may not help and may even be deleterious.
- All patients with a new diagnosis of cardiomyopathy require cardiologic referral.
- Cardiotoxicity is one of the most serious side effects of cancer therapy; cardiac function must be assessed at baseline and during therapy.
- Timely detection and treatment of cardiac and non-cardiac factors that may worsen HF, and in some cases preventative measures, constitute an inherent part of modern HF management.

Key references

Chen MH, Kerkelä R, Force T. Mechanisms of cardiac dysfunction associated with tyrosine kinase inhibitor cancer therapeutics. *Circulation* 2008;118:84–95.

Drazner MH. The progression of hypertensive heart disease. *Circulation* 2011;123:327–34.

Felker GM, Shaw LK, O'Connor CM. A standardized definition of ischemic cardiomyopathy for use in clinical research. *J Am Coll Cardiol* 2002;39: 210–18.

Gianni M, Dentali F, Grandi AM et al. Apical ballooning syndrome or takotsubo cardiomyopathy: a systematic review. *Eur Heart J* 2006;27:1523–9.

Heart Failure Society of America, Lindenfeld J, Albert NM et al. HFSA 2010 Comprehensive Heart Failure Practice Guideline. *J Card Fail* 2010;16:e1–194. Available at www.heartfailureguideline.org, last accessed 11 July 2012.

Houmsse M, Tyler J, Kalbfleisch S. Supraventricular tachycardia causing heart failure. *Curr Opinion Cardiol* 2011;26:261–9.

Jefferies JL, Towbin JA. Dilated cardiomyopathy. *Lancet* 2010;375:752–62.

Marcus FI, McKenna WJ, Sherrill D et al. Diagnosis of arrhythmogenic right ventricular cardiomyopathy/ dysplasia: proposed modification of the task force criteria. *Circulation* 2010;121:1533–41.

Maron BJ, McKenna WJ, Danielson GK et al. American College of Cardiology/European Society of Cardiology Clinical Expert Consensus Document on Hypertrophic Cardiomyopathy. *Eur Heart J* 2003;24:1965–91.

Maron BJ, Towbin JA, Thiene G et al. Contemporary definitions and classification of the cardiomyopathies: an American Heart Association Scientific Statement from the Council on Clinical Cardiology, Heart Failure and Transplantation Committee; Quality of Care and Outcomes Research and Functional Genomics and Translational Biology Interdisciplinary Working Groups; and Council on Epidemiology and Prevention. *Circulation* 2006;113:1807–16.

Mogensen J, Arbustini E. Restrictive cardiomyopathy. *Curr Opinion Cardiol* 2009;24:214–20.

Picano E, Pibarot P, Lancellotti P et al. The emerging role of exercise testing and stress echocardiography in valvular heart disease. *J Am Coll Cardiol* 2009;54:2251–60.

Ramaraj R, Sorrell VL. Peripartum cardiomyopathy: causes, diagnosis, and treatment. *Cleve Clin J Med* 2009;76: 289–96.

Selvanayagam JB, Hawkins PN, Paul B et al. Evaluation and management of the cardiac amyloid. *J Am Coll Card* 2007;50:2101–10.

Vahanian A, Baumgartner H, Bax J et al. Guidelines on the management of valvular heart disease: the Task Force on the Management of Valvular Heart Disease of the European Society of Cardiology. *Eur Heart J* 2007;28: 230–68.

Watkins H, Ashrafian H, Redwood C. Inherited cardiomyopathies. *N Engl J Med* 2011;364:1643–56.

Zaidi A, Sharma S. The athlete's heart. *Br J Hosp Med (Lond)* 2011;72: 275–81.

4 / Comorbidities

Anemia

Anemia (hemoglobin < 130 g/L in men, and < 120 g/L in women) is common in patients with heart failure (HF). It is associated with poorer outcomes and increased mortality, although whether these associations are causative is a matter of debate. Conversely, the correction of anemia has been shown to improve HF-related symptoms, left ventricular (LV) function and quality of life.

The reported prevalence of anemia varies widely, but approximately 37% of congestive HF patients are affected. Prevalence increases with age and with more advanced signs and symptoms of HF (higher NYHA functional classes – see Table 2.1). Clinical characteristics associated with anemia in the HF population are listed in Table 4.1.

Causes

Iron deficiency in the chronic HF population has a reported prevalence of 5–21%. Iron deficiency may be more prevalent in the HF population because of occult gastrointestinal bleeding related to acetylsalicylic acid (ASA; aspirin) use, reduced iron absorption due to gut edema secondary to right ventricular (RV) failure, and uremic gastritis.

Vitamin B$_{12}$ and folic acid deficiencies are relatively uncommon causes of anemia, but they should be considered in the differential diagnosis of

TABLE 4.1

Clinical characteristics associated with increased risk of anemia in patients with chronic heart failure

• Older age	• Use of ACE inhibitors
• Female sex	• Increased JVP
• Chronic kidney disease	• Peripheral edema
• Cachexia	

ACE, angiotensin-converting enzyme; JVP, jugular venous pressure.

anemia. Serum vitamin B_{12} and folate testing are inexpensive, and treatment of deficiencies is cheap and highly effective.

Anemia of chronic disease is a form of anemia that occurs during chronic illness in response to inflammatory processes. In patients with HF, the hemoglobin level is inversely related to levels of proinflammatory cytokines such as tumor necrosis factor (TNF)-α and soluble TNF receptor, and other markers of inflammation such as C-reactive protein.

Dysfunction of erythropoietin production. Renal dysfunction leads to a decline in erythropoietin production through the loss of erythropoietin-producing cells in the kidney. However, it is unusual to see significant anemia due to renal failure until the glomerular filtration rate (GFR) drops below 20 mL/minute. Activation of the renin–angiotensin system, and the consequent angiotensin-converting enzyme (ACE) inhibition and angiotensin-receptor blockade, also reduces erythropoietin production and causes a modest reduction in hemoglobin.

Investigation. It is still unclear whether anemia in HF represents a marker of disease severity and is therefore a prognostic tool, or whether it is a mediator of poorer outcomes and therefore represents a therapeutic target. However, there is evidence that it can worsen cardiac function and symptoms and that correction improves outcome (although further studies are required). Therefore, anemia should be regarded as an easily identifiable and potentially remediable aspect of the disease (Figure 4.1). Common and reversible causes of anemia such as hematinic deficiencies require exclusion, although the underlying etiology is often multifactorial, with the pentad of chronic renal failure, neurohormonal activation, a proinflammatory cytokine milieu, defective erythropoietin production and defective bone marrow function contributing in varying proportions.

Treatment

Blood transfusion may be appropriate in an acute setting for selected patients with severe anemia. The benefit is rapid correction of anemia, although this must be weighed against the risks of circulatory overload, transfusion-transmitted infection, hemolytic transfusion reactions and the longer-term issues of alloimmunization and iron overload.

Iron supplementation and investigation for the underlying cause of the deficiency are indicated when frank iron-deficiency anemia is diagnosed.

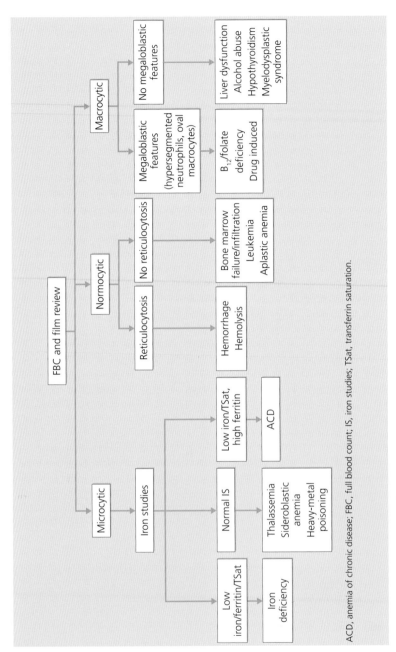

Figure 4.1 An approach to the assessment of anemia using red blood cell size and reticulocyte count to guide investigations.

However, functional iron deficiency associated with elevated inflammatory markers (i.e. anemia of chronic disease) is characterized by adequate iron stores but reduced availability of tissue iron stores for erythropoiesis. Recently, intravenous iron replacement has been shown to improve symptoms, quality of life and exercise capacity in iron-deficient patients with chronic HF.

Erythropoiesis-stimulating agents (ESAs). Trials of ESAs have shown an increased risk of thrombosis in patients with chronic kidney disease (and increased all-cause mortality in trials of patients with malignancy). Therefore, these agents are not recommended as therapy. The exception is in cases of decreased endogenous erythropoietin production due to chronic renal failure.

Pulmonary disease

Chronic obstructive pulmonary disease (COPD) is a common comorbidity in patients with HF, with a prevalence of 10–46%. Conversely, up to 20% of patients with COPD may have undiagnosed HF and up to 40% may have evidence of some LV systolic dysfunction. Cigarette smoking is strongly associated with COPD and coronary artery disease (CAD). It also increases the risk of developing HF by 50%.

Low-grade systemic inflammation is common in patients with COPD and vascular disease, so their coexistence accelerates atherosclerosis and contributes to the increase in adverse cardiovascular events. Furthermore, a reduction in forced expiratory volume in 1 second (FEV_1) in patients with COPD independently predicts cardiovascular mortality even after adjusting for conventional cardiovascular risk factors such as age, cigarette smoking, hypertension, cholesterol and obesity. In patients with HF, COPD increases non-cardiovascular mortality and the overall hospitalization rate.

Diagnosis of one disease in the presence of another is complicated by common symptoms and similar clinical signs, resulting in decreased sensitivity of diagnostic tests such as chest X-ray and ECG.

Natriuretic peptides (type B natriuretic peptide [BNP] and N-terminal hormone of BNP [NT-proBNP]) are produced in response to intracardiac stretch. In patients with dyspnea, normal serum levels of natriuretic peptides (BNP < 100 pg/mL) have high negative predictive value and help to rule out LV systolic dysfunction as a cause of symptoms. Unfortunately, 49 patients with advanced COPD and cor pulmonale often display mild elevation in natriuretic peptide levels.

Echocardiography may provide limited results in up to 50% of patients in view of technical difficulties (poor acoustic windows and endocardial definitions). However, it still remains the initial diagnostic test.

Lung function testing. Airflow obstruction is common in patients with decompensated HF, sometimes resulting in the misdiagnosis and overestimation of COPD severity. With diuresis, mean FEV_1 improves and may even return to normal. Lung function tests should therefore be performed in clinically stable patients without significant pulmonary congestion. Restrictive ventilatory defects are frequent in patients with compensated HF. They mask hyperinflation and obscure diagnosis of COPD in patients with HF.

Prevention and treatment. Respiratory infections are associated with HF decompensation in 10–16% of admissions. Pneumococcal and influenza A vaccinations of elderly patients with HF reduce the rate of hospitalization and associated costs.

In general, concomitant pulmonary and HF therapy is safe, although short-acting β_2-adrenoreceptor agonists and digoxin have potentially negative effects on cardiac and pulmonary function, respectively. Cardioselective beta-blocking agents should not be withheld from COPD patients as no relevant long-term effects on pulmonary function have been established.

Sleep-disordered breathing in the form of obstructive (OSA) or central sleep apnea (CSA) is common in patients with HF (affecting 40–70% of patients).

The effect of sleep-disordered breathing on the cardiovascular system has been an area of intense research. In general, sleep-disordered breathing acts via several independent mechanisms:
- physiological
- increased sympathetic drive
- endothelial dysfunction
- inflammatory effects – an increase in *NFKB1* transcription
- procoagulant effect.

The physiological effects of an exaggerated, negative intrathoracic pressure include an increase in RV preload and a decrease in LV preload with resulting reduction in LV stroke volume. There is also a concomitant decrease in afterload and LV diastolic relaxation. Intermittent elevation of blood pressure accompanying recurrent episodes of apnea and arousal may lead to the development of arterial hypertension. Hypoxia caused by recurrent apnea increases oxidative stress and contributes to further endothelial dysfunction and inflammation. Episodes of inappropriate sinus tachycardia, and atrial and ventricular arrhythmias are common.

Diagnosis. Patients with HF have fewer symptoms of sleep apnea than matched community controls without a cardiac condition, and the two conditions may produce similar symptoms, sometimes leading to delayed diagnosis and treatment of the apnea. Referral for polysomnography should be triggered by a combination of:

- suspicious symptoms (snoring, apnea, unrefreshing sleep, hypersomnolence)
- high-risk clinical features (male, middle aged or older, obese)
- severe underlying cardiomyopathy (LV ejection fraction [LVEF] < 25%)
- willingness to consider treatment.

Prognosis. Untreated sleep-disordered breathing is associated with higher cardiovascular mortality. Moderate-to-severe OSA (apnea-hypopnea index [AHI] > 15) in patients with ischemic cardiomyopathy has been shown to be independently associated with increased mortality (mainly due to sudden cardiac death). A similar association has not been observed in patients without cardiac ischemia. Higher mortality (median survival reduced by 50%) has also been reported in patients with severe LV dysfunction (LVEF < 40%) and CSA.

Treatment. Comprehensive HF therapy with optimal beta-blocker doses is particularly important. Patients with HF and sleep-disordered breathing treated with beta-blockers have a lower prevalence of CSA and a lower AHI, with the dose inversely related to the number of events. Therapy for sleep-disordered breathing in patients with HF may include:

- oxygen
- continuous positive airway pressure (CPAP)
- bi-level ventilation
- servo-adaptive ventilation (in patients with predominant CSA).

Treatment with CPAP alleviates episodes of OSA and associated physiological consequences that may lead to a reduction in LV afterload and ongoing oxidative stress. However, up to 30% of patients may not be able to tolerate it. Evidence that CPAP has a positive effect on cardiovascular morbidity and mortality in patients with HF is lacking, despite observational studies reporting a decrease in sympathetic nervous activity, blood pressure and improvement in cardiac performance (LVEF). Hence, the current indications for CPAP in patients with HF and sleep-disordered breathing are limited to management of diurnal hypersomnolence.

Renal disease

Renal dysfunction is frequently found in patients hospitalized with HF and is strongly associated with increased morbidity and mortality. Additionally, up to 50% of ambulatory patients with stable HF have some degree of renal dysfunction. Moderate to severe renal dysfunction in patients with HF increases the relative mortality risk by 100% (absolute risk > 50% at 5 years). In patients with baseline estimated GFR < 50 mL/min/m² a further drop of 10 mL/min/m² increases mortality by 7%.

It is generally accepted that renal dysfunction is a marker of progressive HF. However, it has also been postulated that renal dysfunction may directly affect the biology of HF by upregulating the renin–angiotensin–aldosterone and sympathetic nervous systems, increasing production of proinflammatory factors and worsening anemia, leading to LV hypertrophy and impaired myocardial contractility.

Cardiorenal syndrome. The existence of both HF and renal dysfunction in an individual is called cardiorenal syndrome (CRS), which is divided into five types, according to the presentation (acute versus chronic) and primary cause of the syndrome (cardiac versus renal):
- CRS type 1 (acute) – acute decompensated HF leading to acute kidney injury (AKI)
- CRS type 2 (chronic) – chronic HF leading to chronic kidney disease
- CRS type 3 (acute renocardiac syndrome) – AKI leading to acute cardiac dysfunction (HF, arrhythmia or coronary ischemia)
- CRS type 4 (chronic renocardiac syndrome) – chronic kidney disease contributing to cardiac dysfunction
- CRS type 5 (secondary CRS) – combined heart and kidney dysfunction due to an acute (e.g. sepsis) or chronic (e.g. diabetes mellitus) systemic disorder.

Therapy differs for the types. In general, careful patient selection and monitoring are crucial. ACE inhibitors or angiotensin-receptor blockers (ARBs) are safe to introduce in patients with CRS type 1 provided the initial rises in serum creatinine and potassium are less than 30% and 5.6 mmol/L, respectively. These drugs should not be initiated in patients with CRS type 3 or known bilateral renal artery stenosis. Chronic therapy with ACE inhibitors or ARBs should be continued (in CRS types 1, 2, 3 and 4), but with close monitoring of serum creatinine and potassium levels.

Beta-blockers should not be initiated in CRS type 1 as they may precipitate an acute drop in cardiac output and a worsening of both AKI and HF, but their continuous use in CRS types 2, 3 and 4 should not be interrupted.

In CRS type 5, the source of infection should be treated (antibiotics, surgery) and supportive cardiac therapy given, including judicious use of intravenous fluids, vasopressors and inotropic agents. If required, hemofiltration may be preferable to hemodialysis, as the latter may cause shifts in intravascular volume, hypotension, arrhythmia and worsening cardiac function.

Liver disease

Transient abnormalities in liver function tests are relatively common in patients with chronic congestive HF. Elevations in aspartate transaminase (AST), alanine transaminase (ALT) and lactate dehydrogenase (LDH), and rarely an increase in serum bilirubin level, have been found on testing. Progression to end-stage liver disease is rare.

Congestive hepatopathy or 'cardiac cirrhosis' is caused by a long-standing elevation in right atrial pressure, as seen in right-sided HF, constrictive pericarditis, pulmonary hypertension and tricuspid valve disease. The primary mechanism of congestive hepatopathy is persistent venous stasis, which leads to hepatic necrosis and fibrosis.

Patients with congestive hepatopathy may develop right upper quadrant pain, anorexia, nausea or vomiting, but the symptoms and signs of HF dominate the disorder. Ascites is a frequent finding. Splenomegaly, jaundice and progression to encephalopathy are rare. Elevations in AST, ALT and serum bilirubin, and prolonged prothrombin time are frequently found on testing. Protein-losing enteropathy with serum hypoalbuminemia may coexist.

The differential diagnoses include alcoholic liver disease, Budd–Chiari syndrome and hepatic vein thrombosis. The effect of congestive hepatopathy on morbidity and mortality is uncertain.

There is no specific therapy except the treatment of the underlying cardiac condition.

Acute ischemic hepatitis has been reported in patients with acute cardiac dysfunction (either new or decompensated chronic HF). It develops in response to a sudden drop in hepatic perfusion resulting from a combination of poor cardiac output and venous congestion.

The condition is characterized by acute hepatocellular necrosis with an increase in serum AST and ALT levels (frequently in the thousands) with accompanying signs (cold periphery, poor urine output, pulmonary congestion) and symptoms (dyspnea, fatigue, nausea, poor appetite) of a low-output state. The synthetic function of the liver is usually retained. The condition is usually subclinical, does not affect the prognosis and improves when cardiac function is restored.

Cirrhotic cardiomyopathy may occur in patients with hepatic cirrhosis; it should be suspected in patients with worsening hemodynamic status. Cardiac involvement is mainly subclinical, long standing and generally well tolerated. The elevated cardiac output often found in patients with cirrhosis is caused by splanchnic arterial vasodilatation, which results in vascular redistribution and a decrease in cardiac preload (despite intravascular volume expansion). Vascular remodeling, with increased vascular compliance and autonomic dysfunction, has also been reported.

The molecular abnormalities associated with cirrhosis, and the negative effect of mediators of cirrhosis (carbon monoxide, endogenous cannabinoids, nitric oxide and proapoptotic kinases) impact on cardiac physiology (QT prolongation, electrical and mechanical dyssynchrony, inotropic and chronotropic incompetence) and may result in diastolic and systolic cardiac dysfunction. The decompensation of cirrhotic cardiomyopathy may be triggered by a sudden change in volume status (i.e. an increase in preload) and vascular resistance (during sepsis, paracentesis, porto–systemic shunt or transplantation).

No specific treatment or management strategies exist for patients with cirrhotic cardiomyopathy, but they should be aggressively monitored during procedures likely to cause decompensation.

Depression

The illness is fairly common among patients with HF, with a reported prevalence of 10–25% in outpatients and 35–70% in inpatients. Most patients have mild symptoms, with fewer than 20% experiencing moderate or severe depression. Women are more likely to be affected by depression than men. The prevalence of depression is inversely related to the severity of HF (NYHA class).

Interestingly, patients with major depression are twice as likely to develop clinical HF over the course of their illness compared with patients without a mood disorder. A stronger risk was found in depressed patients with systolic hypertension.

Prognosis. Depression is associated with non-adherence to medications, poor health-seeking behavior and low social support. It is therefore not unexpected that depression in patients with HF is independently associated with poor prognosis, increased mortality and readmissions to hospital, and use of more medical resources.

In one study, the presence of depression doubled the risk of death and emergency department presentations and increased the total healthcare costs by 29%.

Mechanisms. There are several proposed mechanisms by which depression leads to clinical deterioration and results in worse outcomes in patients with HF. They include:
- neurohormonal activation
- rhythm disturbances
- inflammation
- hypercoagulability
- poor patient adherence
- low social support.

Diagnosis. Initial screening in patients with HF may include the two questions from the Patient Health Questionnaire (PHQ)-2: 'Over the

55

past 2 weeks, how often have you been bothered by (1) little interest or pleasure in doing things, or (2) feeling down, depressed or hopeless?' If the patient answers yes to either part then further assessment with the PHQ-9 is indicated. A score of 10 or more on the questionnaire dictates the need for therapy and specialist assessment (psychologist, psychiatrist).

Treatment. In general, therapeutic intervention in patients with depression and HF includes the combination of an antidepressant (selective serotonin receptor inhibitor such as sertraline), social support and psychotherapy.

Key points – comorbidities

- Patients with heart failure (HF) should undergo regular monitoring for early diagnosis of anemia and appropriate investigation to determine the cause. Therapeutic intervention should be tailored to the individual, taking into account the velocity of hemoglobin fall, the presence or absence of concomitant renal dysfunction and the cause of the anemia.
- Despite inherent diagnostic limitations it is important for clinicians to establish the presence of pulmonary disease and to introduce early therapy for both chronic obstructive pulmonary disease and HF in order to limit their negative impact on morbidity and mortality.
- Early diagnosis of sleep-disordered breathing is important as treatment with continuous positive airway pressure in symptomatic patients is effective.
- HF therapy is challenging in the context of comorbid renal disease, as vasodilators may precipitate an increase in serum creatinine and potassium levels; however, current evidence supports the use of these drugs in patients with CRS type 1 providing the initial increase in serum creatinine and potassium are less than 30% and 5.6 mmol/L, respectively.
- Acute ischemic hepatitis may develop in HF with low-output state and is generally reversible.
- Clinical depression is not uncommon in patients with HF and is associated with a marked increase in HF morbidity and mortality.

Key references

Anand IS. Anemia and chronic heart failure implications and treatment options. *J Am Coll Cardiol* 2008;52:501–11.

Anand IS, Kuskowski MA, Rector TS et al. Anemia and change in hemoglobin over time related to mortality and morbidity in patients with chronic heart failure: results from Val-HeFT. *Circulation* 2005;112: 1121–7.

Bohlius J, Schmidlin K, Brillant C et al. Recombinant human erythropoiesis-stimulating agents and mortality in patients with cancer: a meta-analysis of randomised trials. *Lancet* 2009;373:1532–42.

Glassman A, Maj MM, Sartorius N, eds. *Depression and Heart Disease.* Chichester: Wiley-Blackwell, 2011.

Groenveld HF, Januzzi JL, Damman K et al. Anemia and mortality in heart failure patients a systematic review and meta-analysis. *J Am Coll Cardiol* 2008;52:818–27.

Hawkins NM, Petrie MC, Jhund PS et al. Heart failure and chronic obstructive pulmonary disease: diagnostic pitfalls and epidemiology. *Eur J Heart Fail* 2009;11:130–9.

Ishani A, Weinhandl E, Zhao Z et al. Angiotensin-converting enzyme inhibitor as a risk factor for the development of anemia, and the impact of incident anemia on mortality in patients with left ventricular dysfunction. *J Am Coll Cardiol* 2005;45:391–9.

Kasai T, Bradley TD. Obstructive sleep apnea and heart failure: pathophysiologic and therapeutic implications. *J Am Coll Cardiol* 2011;57:119–27.

McGonigle RJ, Wallin JD, Shadduck RK, Fisher JW. Erythropoietin deficiency and inhibition of erythropoiesis in renal insufficiency. *Kidney Int* 1984;25:437–44.

Palmer SC, Navaneethan SD, Craig JC et al. Meta-analysis: erythropoiesis-stimulating agents in patients with chronic kidney disease. *Ann Intern Med* 2010;153:23–33.

Rauchhaus M, Doehner W, Francis DP et al. Plasma cytokine parameters and mortality in patients with chronic heart failure. *Circulation* 2000;102:3060–7.

Ronco C, Haapio M, House AA et al. Cardiorenal syndrome. *J Am Coll Cardiol* 2008;52:1527–39.

Tang WH, Tong W, Jain A et al. Evaluation and long-term prognosis of new-onset, transient, and persistent anemia in ambulatory patients with chronic heart failure. *J Am Coll Cardiol* 2008;51:569–76.

Case history

A 67-year-old man with diabetes mellitus, hypertension and renal impairment is referred to the cardiology outpatient department because of fatigue. He is overweight and relatively inactive, but still able to visit his country property and went hunting as recently as last year. He has experienced shortness of breath when climbing two flights of stairs at home and has difficulty in walking uphill to his house. He has no history of ischemic heart disease or other cardiac symptoms. His blood pressure is 164/96 mmHg and he has an irregular pulse of 102 beats per minute. He has no jugular venous distension or edema, and his chest is clear to auscultation; the apex beat is impalpable but there is a blowing pansystolic murmur at the apex. The chest X-ray shows cardiomegaly and the ECG shows atrial fibrillation with left bundle branch block.

This is a typical presentation of decompensating chronic heart failure (HF). The following questions need to be asked:

- Is this really HF?
- What was the functional status before this deterioration?
- What is the ejection fraction?
- What is the underlying etiology?
- What is the precipitant of this exacerbation?
- Is there coronary artery disease?
- What social support is in place that will support care at home?
- Are there features that may eventually require device therapy (implantable cardiac defibrillator [ICD] or cardiac resynchronization therapy [CRT])?

Table 5.1 provides an overview of the factors that contribute to acute presentations.

Symptoms and signs

The onset of HF symptoms (Table 5.2) may be acute (typically with pulmonary edema, even with cardiogenic shock) or subacute. Both right and left HF may occur in the context of low output (fatigue, syncope and hypotension), and both right- and left-sided HF usually occur together.

TABLE 5.1

Factors that contribute to acute presentation of heart failure

- Poor adherence
  - medication
  - sodium/water restriction
  - obesity
  - alcohol
- Pharmacotherapeutic issues
  - failure to use/inadequate dosing/too rapid introduction of beta-blockers and vasodilators
  - ineffective diuretic prescription
  - use of potentially harmful medications (antiarrhythmics, NSAIDs)
- Inadequate syndrome recognition
- Inadequate control of hypertension, diabetes mellitus
- Failure to correct areas of reversible myocardial ischemia or surgery including valve repair/replacement or aneurysmectomy
- Unrecognized hypo- or hyperthyroidism
- Cardiovascular deconditioning
- Failure to correct or control atrial fibrillation

NSAID, non-steroidal anti-inflammatory drug.

Assessment of functional class (see Table 2.1), based on exercise capacity, is important in chronic HF because it is linked to outcome – the annualized mortality in NYHA class IV HF is approximately 50%, which is four to five times that of class II and twice that of class III.

The signs of HF are often subtle. Jugular venous pressure is a sign of intravascular volume overload that is often overlooked (25–58% of cases) (Table 5.3).

The Framingham criteria for HF are shown in Table 5.4. However, these features are ill-suited to the recognition of HF with preserved ejection fraction, and the European Society of Cardiology (ESC) has proposed the incorporation of imaging findings in order to facilitate the recognition of HF in patients presenting with exercise intolerance alone (see Table 5.4).

59

TABLE 5.2

Symptoms of heart failure

Left-sided	Right-sided
• Exertional dyspnea	• Edema
• Orthopnea	• Abdominal distension (due to ascites)
• Paroxysmal nocturnal dyspnea	
	• Right upper quadrant discomfort (due to liver congestion)

TABLE 5.3

Jugular venous pressure

• Changes with respiration (usually decreases with deep inspiration)

• Multiphasic pulsation (the JVP 'beats' twice in a cardiac cycle [Figure 5.1], while the carotid artery only has one beat)

• Location (but not height) changes with alteration of posture. Measurement is taken from the xiphisternum. The normal JVP will not be seen if the patient is lying flat (the vein is distended) or sitting up (the vein is empty). A 45° tilt is the best starting position, but if JVP is not apparent, sit the patient up further or lie them down further. The location of the pulse varies with the angle of the neck (Figure 5.2). *You must see the upper limit of the JVP*

• Remove pulsation with venous compression (the JVP can be stopped by lightly pressing against the neck; it will fill from above)

• Hepatojugular reflux (firm but gentle pressure over the right upper quadrant will move blood from the splanchnic to the central veins). Failure to distend the jugular veins indicates they may already be filled. Typically, distension is persistent in HF

HF, heart failure; JVP, jugular venous pressure.

Acute heart failure

The initial clinical picture of acute HF reflects the varying degree of impairment of cardiac output and elevation in LV diastolic pressure or pulmonary artery wedge pressure (obtained at left and right heart

catheterization, respectively).

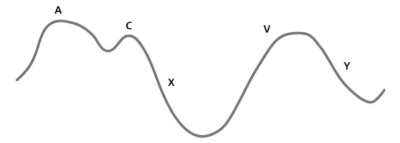

Figure 5.1 The multiphasic wave form of jugular venous pulsation. A, atrial contraction ending in synchrony with the carotid artery pulse. C, right ventricular contraction causing the tricuspid valve to bulge towards the right atrium. X, atrial relaxation and filling. V, venous filling when the tricuspid valve is closed (during and after the carotid pulse). Prominent v waves indicate tricuspid regurgitation. Y, rapid emptying of the atrium after the tricuspid valve opens.

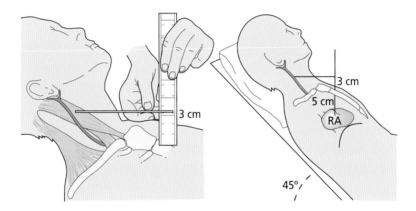

Figure 5.2 To visually assess the jugular venous pressure (JVP), position the patient at 45° (or at an angle between supine and upright where the venous pulse can be detected), with the head turned slightly to the side; this allows the viewer to profile the pulsation against the contour of the neck. Place a ruler vertically from the horizontal plane of the sternal angle, then use another straight edge to create a horizontal line from the visible pulsation of the jugular vein. The location of the pulse varies with the angle of the neck, so it is important to find the upper limit of the JVP. The upper normal limit is 3 cm; as the right atrium (RA) is 5 cm below the sternal angle in most individuals, normal JVP is described as less than 8 cmH$_2$O.

61

TABLE 5.4

Criteria for heart failure

Framingham: requires the simultaneous presence of at least two major criteria or one major criterion in conjunction with two minor criteria:

Major criteria
- Nocturnal dyspnea
- Venous distension/hepatojugular reflux (see Table 5.3)
- Crackles or pulmonary edema
- Cardiomegaly on chest radiography
- S3 gallop (a third heart sound)

Minor criteria
- Tachycardia
- Bilateral ankle edema
- Exertional dyspnea
- Nocturnal cough
- Hepatomegaly
- Reduction of vital capacity

European Society for Cardiology:
Essential features
Symptoms of HF (e.g. dyspnea, fatigue, ankle swelling)
Objective evidence of cardiac dysfunction (at rest)

Non-essential features
In cases where the diagnosis is in doubt: evidence of a response to HF treatment

Patients with acute HF can present with one of several distinct hemodynamic profiles, based on the degree of pulmonary congestion (wet versus dry) and the state of tissue perfusion (warm versus cold) (Figure 5.3).

More specific for acute HF is Gheorgiade's classification in which the therapeutic target – cardiac output, blood pressure or intravascular volume – dictates the intervention.

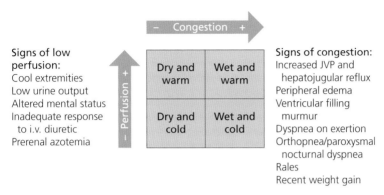

Figure 5.3 Hemodynamic clinical profiles of acute heart failure. i.v., intravenous; JVP, jugular venous pressure.

Arrhythmias

Arrhythmias may play a part in both acute and chronic HF. Atrial fibrillation is an important precipitant of acute deterioration and is itself engendered by persistent elevation of filling pressure leading to left atrial enlargement. Atrial arrhythmias contribute to reduced functional capacity, as atrial systole makes an important contribution to stroke volume, especially in the context of LV filling problems and particularly with exercise. Although some patients die from progressive HF, ventricular arrhythmias are an important cause of death in patients with HF. The risk of fatal arrhythmias is greatest in the presence of low ejection fraction, but because of the higher number of patients with less severe reduction of ejection fraction, this group has the highest absolute number of sudden deaths.

Investigations

Blood tests. In most patients, routine biochemistry includes blood tests for electrolytes and renal and liver function, a full blood count (to assess anemia) and evaluation of C-reactive protein levels if infection is suspected. Thyroid function tests and iron studies should be obtained at initial presentation in patients with cardiomyopathies. Type B natriuretic peptide (BNP) levels need only be assessed when echocardiography is not available and the diagnosis is in doubt.

Electrocardiography will help to identify atrial fibrillation, evidence of CAD or LV hypertrophy and conduction delay or abnormalities (e.g. QT_c interval).

Chest X-rays can be used to identify pulmonary congestion or chamber enlargement.

Echocardiography. An echocardiogram is appropriate at original diagnosis or if the patient deteriorates. The main goals of echocardiography are to assess LV size, systolic and diastolic LV function, disturbances of regional function (which suggest an ischemic heart disease etiology), valve regurgitation and LV hypertrophy. Patients with HF who undergo echocardiography have significantly better outcomes than those who do not – presumably because of the initiation of appropriate therapy.

Cardiac magnetic resonance imaging (CMR). There are three major indications for CMR in HF:
- to supplement poor quality echocardiographic images (often due to obesity or chronic lung disease)
- to obtain accurate measurements when the echo results are ambiguous (e.g. ejection fraction < 35% has specific implications for device therapy)
- to assess myocardial scar burden.

The last is used to detect and quantify transmural scarring in CAD (see assessment of viability, below) and to identify scarring in non-coronary heart disease.

CMR has greater capability for tissue characterization than echocardiography, and may be used to identify specific etiologies for HF, some of which have clear prognostic or therapeutic implications (e.g. amyloidosis, sarcoidosis), while others are less certain (e.g. myocarditis). The use of CMR in HF is extremely variable between centers.

Imaging for coronary disease and viable myocardium. The role of CAD should be considered in any patient with HF. Coronary investigation is often not indicated in young patients for whom there is a good alternative explanation for their symptoms; however, most patients with HF are elderly and in these patients coronary angiography may be considered if it is felt that the patient is a suitable candidate for a revascularization procedure. Coronary CT has been used in these circumstances, although calcification, which may preclude recognition of stenosis, should be expected in older patients.

Once coronary disease has been identified, the next question is whether this is an 'innocent bystander'. A variety of tests have been reported for the detection of viable myocardium, ranging from the simple (single-photon-emission CT, dobutamine echo) to the complex (MRI, positron emission tomography). Although the recently reported STICH trial found no relationship between the results of viability imaging and outcome, it is important to consider not only the presence of dysfunctional but viable tissue, but also its extent, i.e. the total burden of compromised myocardium, including ischemia.

Functional testing involves exercise testing using either a treadmill or ergometer, with or without analysis of expired gases to obtain peak oxygen consumption or carbon dioxide generation. Functional testing is of value for objective quantification of exercise capacity at any stage, but especially in patients who are being evaluated for advanced therapies, including devices and transplantation.

Key points – diagnosis

- Assessment of functional class, based on exercise capacity, is important in chronic heart failure (HF) as it is linked to outcome.
- Also key to the diagnosis of HF is the assessment of ejection fraction, underlying etiology and precipitating factors, and the role of coronary artery disease.
- The hemodynamic profile of acute HF varies according to the degree of pulmonary congestion (wet versus dry) and the state of tissue perfusion (warm versus cold).
- Atrial arrhythmias contribute to a reduction in functional capacity, while ventricular arrhythmias are an important cause of death in HF patients.
- Investigations in HF patients include blood tests, ECG, chest X-ray, echocardiography and other imaging techniques.
- Functional testing is of particular value in patients deemed suitable candidates for devices or transplantation.

Key references

Ho KK, Anderson KM, Kannel WB et al. Survival after the onset of congestive heart failure in Framingham Heart Study subjects. *Circulation* 1993;88:107–15.

Paulus WJ, Tschöpe C, Sanderson JE et al. How to diagnose diastolic heart failure: a consensus statement on the diagnosis of heart failure with normal left ventricular ejection fraction by the Heart Failure and Echocardiography Associations of the European Society of Cardiology. *Eur Heart J* 2007;28: 2539–50.

Multidisciplinary strategies

The cost of managing patients with heart failure (HF) is substantial and continues to grow, with the main area of expenditure being high rehospitalization rates (see Chapter 1). In order to improve patient care and reduce healthcare costs, multidisciplinary HF management programs have been designed for patients with severe symptomatic HF, which unify and coordinate their care throughout their illness and within the various service-delivery systems (i.e. the hospital, outpatient clinic and community setting). The mode of intervention varies from direct face-to-face contact to telephone consultation and the use of telemedicine. In general, management programs do not include diagnosed patients with mild symptoms (no effect on outcomes), those with HF and preserved systolic function (no available evidence) or severely ill patients at the end stage of the disease (in need of a palliative care approach – see Chapter 9).

Integral to all HF management programs are:
• prompt assessment of disease activity and the interventions required
• supervised medical treatment, including drug titration
• improved access to care
• comprehensive patient education
• psychosocial support.

Most programs involve nurses and physicians specialized in HF. Input from pharmacists, allied health staff (physiotherapists, occupational therapists, nutritionists, social workers) or psychologists varies; some of the programs incorporate all of these services.

Effectiveness. The available evidence suggests the following.
• Strategies that incorporate follow-up by a specialized multidisciplinary team (either in a clinic or non-clinic setting) reduce mortality, HF hospitalizations and all-cause hospitalizations.
• Programs that focus on enhancing patient self-care activities reduce HF hospitalizations and all-cause hospitalizations but have no effect on mortality.

- Strategies that employ telephone contact and advise patients to attend their primary care physician in the event of deterioration reduce HF hospitalizations but not mortality or all-cause hospitalizations.
- Remote monitoring programs (including telemonitoring or structured telephone support – see below) reduce the rates of admission to hospital for chronic HF and all-cause mortality.
- Most of the programs are cost-effective or cost-neutral.

Telemonitoring and telehomecare. Keeping patients in their own environment is preferable, and the use of telehomecare (follow-up by telephone) and telemonitoring (using wireless technology) has been developed with this aim in mind. Information such as daily weight, heart rate, blood pressure and adherence to treatment can be assessed over the telephone or transmitted wirelessly to allow rapid and serial review. The results from a number of studies looking at both intensive home-care assessment and remote analysis have been variable. In a recent Cochrane review of 25 studies involving more than 8000 patients, telemonitoring significantly reduced mortality and HF rehospitalization. However, other studies have indicated more neutral outcomes and, overall, current evidence does not support a strong effect on patient outcomes.

Although implantable devices, such as pacemakers and defibrillators, are capable of providing real-time information on a daily basis, such as heart-rate variability, patient-activity status and assessment of lung fluid volume, they have yet to provide sufficiently accurate predictive data. Newer devices currently under intensive study may be able to monitor hemodynamic changes either directly (left atrial pressures) or indirectly (via the pulmonary circulation or by transthoracic or intracardiac impedance). Early signs are promising but there is still too great a variation in outcome for results to be predictive.

General principles of non-pharmacological management

General non-pharmacological management may be as important as the prescription of HF-specific medications. The majority of HF care is conducted in the home by either the patient and/or the caregiver. It is therefore essential that all HF patients and those who care for them receive comprehensive education and counseling to develop the knowledge, skills, strategies, problem-solving approaches and motivation required to adhere to a complex treatment plan and effectively participate in HF self-care. It is important to include carers and family members in this education as HF patients often experience difficulties with cognition, functional ability and other conditions that may limit their understanding of what is required. Non-adherence to HF management plans can be related to patient and/or caregiver misconceptions and lack of knowledge.

Self-care involves active participation in the maintenance and management of HF. Included within self-care maintenance are healthy lifestyle choices, treatment adherence and monitoring of behaviors. Self-care management is a cognitive process that involves the recognition of signs and symptoms of worsening HF, evaluation of the importance of a change in symptoms, implementation of a self-care strategy (such as increasing diuretic medication) and evaluating the effectiveness of any changes.

Education should be structured and individualized to the patient's specific situation (e.g. literacy level, cultural background) (Table 6.1).

Treatment adherence. Although good adherence to HF management regimens is associated with a decrease in morbidity and mortality, and improvement in wellbeing, only 20–60% of patients with HF adhere to their prescribed medical and non-medical treatment plan. It has been demonstrated that some patients either misunderstand or have trouble recalling information provided on HF self-management (such as instructions on dietary changes).

In order to promote increased adherence for patients with HF, the following are recommended:
- a strong relationship between the healthcare team and patients
- adequate social support and participation by the family in education programs and decisions regarding treatment and care
- provision of adequate knowledge of all aspects of treatment including effects, side effects and titration of medications.

Symptom recognition. Breathlessness and fatigue are classic symptoms of HF and are often used to determine progression of the condition. Other, less commonly documented, symptoms include dizziness, loss of appetite, increased satiety, peripheral edema, abdominal swelling, bloating or

TABLE 6.1

Components of self-care education

- Understanding the pathology and treatment of heart failure, the underlying condition and comorbidities
- Understanding the importance of adherence to pharmacological and non-pharmacological treatments and beneficial lifestyle modifications
- Monitoring own condition and recognizing deterioration
- Seeking assistance when signs and symptoms worsen
- Understanding the function of the medication and possible side effects
- Inclusion of family, friends and caregivers as part of the educational intervention
- Use of a skills-based approach rather than only providing information (e.g. demonstration on how to read sodium content on a food label)
- Use of multimedia resources (DVDs, books, brochures, verbal education, support groups, computer-based programs)

discomfort, persistent cough, paroxysmal nocturnal dyspnea and palpitations. The clinician should evaluate the symptom(s) objectively and recognize their importance to the affected individual.

Patients and /or caregivers should understand the variable nature of HF symptoms and learn to recognize decompensation warning symptoms early in order to take appropriate action.

Weight monitoring, and fluid and sodium management. The maintenance of a normal blood volume is paramount in the management of HF. Increases in bodyweight are often associated with fluid retention and therefore deterioration in HF and possible hospital admission. The management of volume overload in HF patients frequently requires intravenous diuretics and modification to fluid and sodium intake. However, hypovolemia due to increased fluid loss from diarrhea, vomiting or overuse of diuretics, or insufficient fluid intake, brings different but equally debilitating symptoms such as hypotension, electrolyte disturbances and changes to renal function.

Patients should be encouraged to weigh themselves daily, each morning after emptying their bladder, in order to detect either rapid weight gain, which might indicate they are retaining too much fluid, or rapid weight loss of a similar amount in the same period, which might indicate dehydration. Ideally, these weights should be recorded in a weight diary so that trends can be monitored over time. This is also advantageous to those with cognitive impairment. Patients and their carers should be instructed to contact their healthcare practitioner or HF nurse if weight increases or decreases unexpectedly by more than 2 kg over 2 or 3 consecutive days as they may need further assessment or a change to their diuretic regimen.

If patients have demonstrated the ability to self-care, it may be appropriate for them to regulate their own diuretic dose based on daily weight monitoring and assessment of HF symptoms. Initially, the increased dose should be a single multiple of the previous dose (e.g. if the usual dose is 40 mg daily, the increase should be to 80 mg daily) for a period of 3 days or until euvolemia is achieved. If there is no change in status the patient should be encouraged to seek the assistance of the healthcare provider or HF nurse.

Patients with severe symptoms of HF should be encouraged to limit their fluid intake to 1.5–2 L/day (except in warmer weather), particularly if they have associated hyponatremia. There is no evidence to suggest fluid limitation is useful in patients with mild to moderate HF. Excessive dietary sodium intake contributes to fluid overload and is a major cause of preventable admission to hospital. It has been suggested that excessive sodium intake may also contribute to diuretic resistance. When combined with a diuretic regimen, a low-sodium diet can result in beneficial hemodynamic and clinical effects. In patients with mild symptoms, a sodium restriction to 3 g per day is sufficient to control extracellular fluid volume, while those with more severe symptoms should reduce sodium intake to 2 g/day.

Patients should be assessed on their knowledge of sodium content in the foods they consume and then educated on how to identify and measure sodium intake.

Healthy lifestyle choices

Physical activity. Multiple factors contribute to physical deconditioning in patients with HF. Symptoms of effort-related dyspnea and fatigue dominate the clinical picture, thus reducing functional capacity. In general, exercise limitation is caused by a combination of low cardiac output and non-cardiac causes such as peripheral vasoconstriction/endothelial dysfunction, ventilatory limitation and skeletal muscle changes. The presence of multiple medical comorbidities (e.g. depression, sleep-disordered breathing, arthritis) further limits physical performance in this group.

Benefits of regular exercise. Physical activity has been shown to improve functional capacity, symptoms and neurohormonal abnormalities. Provisional evidence also suggests that regular exercise, which is considered a safe and cost-effective intervention, may reduce hospital admissions and improve survival. The benefits of regular exercise in patients with HF include peripheral adaptation of the skeletal muscles and autonomic nervous system, and a significant increase in exercise capacity (by about 15% maximum oxygen consumption [VO_2max]). Exercise also leads to improvement in overall quality-of-life scores.

Contraindications. Regular physical activity is strongly recommended for all medically stable patients with HF unless they are in NYHA class IV or have other limiting symptoms such as angina (Table 6.2). Implantable cardiac defibrillator (ICD) settings must be reviewed before any exercise is undertaken.

Structured exercise programs. All medically stable patients should be considered for a structured, specifically designed exercise and rehabilitation program that incorporates both an aerobic component of low-to-moderate intensity (e.g. walking, cycling) for most days of the week, and strengthening exercises comprising light weights and stretching. Patients should be encouraged to perform 1 to 3 sets of 8 to 12 exercise cycles with weights or 'therabands'. However, to date, research on strength training has been limited.

In general, exercise prescription in patients with HF should include:

- an initial phase of 1:1 duration of exercise versus rest, to be continued until the patient reaches level 3 on the Borg scale (40–50% VO_2max) (Table 6.3)
- an improvement phase of 2:1 duration of exercise versus rest, with the aim of reaching level 4 on the Borg scale (50–80% VO_2max).

If a structured exercise regimen is not possible because of comorbidities or inability to attend, clinically stable patients should be encouraged to keep as active as possible. A regimen of about 20 minutes of exercise at 60–70% of the maximal heart rate (some patients wear heart monitors to

TABLE 6.2

Contraindications to exercise in patients with heart failure

Absolute contraindications

- Progressive worsening of exercise tolerance or dyspnea at rest or on exertion over previous 3–5 days
- Significant ischemia at low exercise intensities (< 2 METs or ~50 Watts)
- Uncontrolled diabetes mellitus
- Acute systemic illness or fever
- Recent embolism
- Thrombophlebitis
- Active pericarditis or myocarditis
- Severe aortic stenosis
- Valvular heart disease requiring surgery
- Myocardial infarction within previous 3 weeks
- New-onset atrial fibrillation
- Resting heart rate > 120 bpm

Relative contraindications

- ≥ 2 kg increase in body mass over previous 1–3 days
- Concurrent continuous or intermittent dobutamine therapy
- > 10 mmHg drop in systolic blood pressure with exercise
- Class IV (NYHA) dyspnea
- Complex ventricular arrhythmia at rest or appearing with exertion
- Supine resting heart rate ≥ 100 bpm
- Pre-existing comorbidities
- Moderate aortic stenosis
- BP > 180/110 mmHg (evaluated on a case-by-case basis)

BP, blood pressure; bpm, beats per minute; MET, metabolic equivalent of task – a physiological measure expressing the energy cost of physical activities (< 3 METs = light exercise/rest, > 6 METs = vigorous exercise); NYHA, New York Heart Association.

TABLE 6.3

Borg scale: rating of perceived exertion

0	Nothing
0.5	Very, very weak
1	Very weak
2	Weak
3	Moderate
4	Somewhat strong
5	Strong
6	
7	Very strong
8	
9	
10	Very, very strong

gauge their level of exertion) or the patient's perceived exertion of 'moderate' three times per week is associated with improved exercise capacity. Referral to an exercise physiologist or physiotherapist is recommended if there is no access to group exercise programs.

The importance of warm-up and cool-down periods must be emphasized in HF patients. A warm-up period of 10–15 minutes reduces the risk of cardiac ischemia, and improves peripheral circulation and oxygen extraction. A prolonged cool-down period after exercise helps to reduce the build up of lactic acid, and damp orthostatic responses to exercise and drug-induced dilated peripheral circulation.

Most of the current exercise programs consist of 12 weeks' supervised exercises with ongoing home-based aerobic training.

Nutrition and weight management. Obesity can increase the risk of developing HF or worsen symptoms. Weight reduction is recommended in the obese (body mass index $\geq$ 30 kg/m^2) in an effort to improve physical activity and quality of life. Saturated fat intake should be limited in all patients with HF and especially those who have concomitant coronary heart disease. See *Fast Facts: Obesity* for more information on weight management.

Subclinical or clinical malnutrition or cardiac cachexia is a common problem in HF patients and contributes to weakness and fatigue. Reduced nutritional intake because of lack of appetite, liver or gut dysfunction, systemic inflammation or activation of neurohormonal mechanisms can lead to cachexia, which is associated with a poor prognosis. Patients who have lost more than 6% of their stable dry weight in the previous 6 months should be assessed for an underlying cause, treated as appropriate and referred to a dietician for nutritional support.

Patients should receive advice on healthy eating to maintain optimal nutrition. This can be achieved through brochures, cookbooks and referral to a dietician.

Smoking is the most important preventable risk factor for developing cardiovascular disease, pulmonary disease and cancer. It is atherogenic, reduces oxygenation of the blood, promotes vasoconstriction, impairs endothelial and respiratory function, and is arrhythmogenic, leading to a reduction in physical performance and worsening of symptoms.

It is strongly recommended that people who smoke should quit. It is safe to employ nicotine replacement and other smoking cessation strategies along with support and advice about stopping smoking (see *Fast Facts: Smoking Cessation*).

Alcohol. Excessive alcohol intake can be a cause of HF. It has the potential to increase the risk of arrhythmias, increase blood pressure and add to the fluid burden of the HF patient. It can also increase body mass due to its high energy load, and may alter the metabolism of some medications used in HF.

Daily intake should be reduced to 10–20 g (one to two standard drinks) per day; patients with suspected alcohol-induced cardiomyopathy should abstain completely. Vitamin supplementation (especially thiamine) should be considered for people with a history of high alcohol consumption and poor nutrition.

Other lifestyle considerations

Sexual activity. It is common for HF patients to experience sexual problems related to cardiovascular disease, medical treatment (beta-blockers, digoxin, spironolactone, thiazide diuretic) or physiological

75

factors such as fatigue and depression. Such problems adversely affect the quality of life of the patient and their partner. There is, however, little evidence related to sexual activity in patients with HF and it has been suggested that sexual activity is likely to be safe. Patients who are able to achieve approximately 6 METs (metabolic equivalents of task [see Table 6.2]) of exercise (i.e. able to climb two flights of stairs without stopping due to angina, breathlessness or fatigue) should be able to undertake regular sexual activity.

It is important to provide sensitive individualized assessment, education and counseling for patients about returning to, or ongoing, sexual function.

Erectile dysfunction (ED) is a common complaint in patients with HF. Therapy should start with optimization of HF. If no improvement is observed, the ED is most likely to be related to medications. In these circumstances, patients may consider avoiding digoxin and thiazide diuretics, changing some medications (spironolactone to eplerenone, beta-blocker to carvedilol) or taking a specific treatment for ED (a phosphodiesterase-5 inhibitor, e.g. sildenafil). Sildenafil is not currently recommended for patients with severe HF (class III–IV symptoms) and is contraindicated if the patient is using a nitrate preparation.

Sleep-disordered breathing (see also Chapter 4), consisting of obstructive or central sleep apnea, can occur in up to 50% of patients with moderate to severe HF and may be associated with increased morbidity and mortality. All patients with moderate to severe HF should be screened for the likely presence of sleep apnea using the Berlin Questionnaire or equivalent, and referred for definitive assessment and treatment if positive.

Lifestyle modification such as smoking cessation, weight reduction and abstinence from alcohol can reduce the risk of sleep-disordered breathing.

Depression. (See also Chapter 4.) The prevalence of depression in patients with HF is significantly higher than in age- and sex-matched controls; approximately 20% of patients with HF also have depression. There is also consistent evidence to support an independent causal association between depression, social isolation and lack of quality social support, and coronary heart disease. Depression is related to a reduction in self-care activities, increased hospitalization and reduced survival.

Although cognitive behavior therapy and selective serotonin-reuptake inhibitors (SSRIs) reduce depression in cardiac patients, there is no evidence of a significant reduction in mortality in this population. SSRIs can increase sodium levels, so patients should be monitored during active treatment.

Immunization. Patients with chronic disease, especially those aged over 65, are particularly vulnerable to the complications of influenza, which could lead to increased morbidity and hospital admissions, and premature death. There are no HF-specific randomized studies of immunization, but studies of immunization in those with cardiovascular disease have shown a reduction in the relative risk of mortality within 1 year. Immunization has no protective effect in younger patients.

Yearly influenza vaccination and vaccination against pneumococcal diseases should be undertaken for patients with symptomatic HF.

Travel for patients with HF is possible but complex, and preparation is the key. Any intention to travel should be discussed with a healthcare practitioner before arrangements are made. Patients wishing to travel to hot and humid destinations should be counseled about the risk of dehydration and adjustments to their fluid-management regimen, while patients with ischemic cardiomyopathy should be warned that colder climates can precipitate angina because of the increase in peripheral vascular resistance. Prophylaxis for deep vein thrombosis (DVT) should be considered in patients preparing for long flights.

Driving. The driving rules for patients with HF vary between countries and clinicians should refer to national guidelines (see Further reading, page 134). In general, patients with a commercial driving license and symptomatic HF are banned from driving. In the UK re/licensing may be permitted provided:

- LV ejection fraction is 40% or higher
- there is no other disqualifying condition.

Exercise or other functional testing may be required depending on the likely cause of the HF. In Australia, for a commercial driving license to be reissued individuals must demonstrate:

- minimal symptomatic status
- satisfactory response to therapy

- recent LVEF above 40% on echocardiography
- no evidence of cardiac ischemia, with exercise tolerance at 90% or greater of age/sex-predicted exercise capacity (according to the Bruce protocol).

Regular assessment with annual testing is advised (Australia).

Air travel may have a negative effect on HF either directly through hypoxia or immobilization, or indirectly and very rarely because of interference of an electromagnetic field, cosmic radiation or vibration with implanted devices such as pacemakers or implantable cardiac defibrillators (ICDs).

During flights, the changes in ambient partial pressure of oxygen (pO_2) due to the changing altitude cause a drop in arterial pO_2 in healthy subjects by about 30% to 62–67 mmHg (8.2–9 kPa). The resulting hypoxia could have negative cardiovascular consequences in HF patients.

Effects of hypoxia in heart failure. Significant hypoxia may have a deleterious effect on patients suffering from LV dysfunction. It can lead to tachycardia or an elevation in systemic and pulmonary blood pressure, and can even trigger arrhythmia or coronary ischemia in patients with underlying coronary artery disease (CAD). However, in patients with HF, pulmonary vasoconstriction may help protect the pulmonary micro-vasculature from increased pressure. It appears that the systemic vascular resistance falls in response to hypoxia (thought to be mediated by nitric oxide), which may limit rises in pulmonary venous and LV filling pressures.

However, there is a lack of convincing evidence. Two studies have shown that in patients with class III–IV NYHA HF with ejection fractions less than 40%, controllable hypoxia increased blood pressure and positive airway pressure, and lowered ventricular filling pressures but did not cause any significant symptoms or change to workload. No changes in blood pressure or dyspnea were noted in patients with NYHA class II HF who were tested during a simulated 7-hour flight.

Acute left ventricular failure. The risk of hospitalization for HF following acute myocardial infarction (MI) is highest in the few weeks after the infarction but stabilizes after 45 days. Once any precipitant has been identified and treated, most patients should be stabilized within 6 weeks and are considered safe to fly.

Chronic heart failure. Passengers with stable chronic HF without recent changes in symptoms or medication are likely to be able to tolerate the mild hypoxia of the aircraft cabin environment even if they have severe HF. However, they should avoid physical exertion at the airport and make sure that they take their regular medication. It is probably prudent for passengers who are severely limited with NYHA class IV symptoms not to fly without special consideration and the availability of in-flight oxygen.

Deep vein thrombosis/venous thromboembolism risk. Patients with HF are at moderate risk of DVT/venous thromboembolism (VTE) while travelling by air. In general, patients should keep mobile, practice regular flexion and extension exercises of the lower limbs, and avoid dehydration. Alcohol and sedatives should be avoided. Compression stockings have been shown to reduce risk in the non-HF population. Prophylactic low-molecular-weight heparin may be considered in patients with severe HF on long intercontinental flights.

Electromagnetic interference. Pacemakers and ICDs are inherently susceptible to electromagnetic interference. In an ICD, electromagnetic interference may be falsely interpreted as tachyarrhythmia and trigger inappropriate therapies (anti-tachycardia pacing or shocks). The risk of electromagnetic interference from metal detectors is remote. The accumulated data suggest that the risk of clinically significant electromagnetic interference affecting pacemakers or ICDs in the airplane environment is minimal.

Cosmic radiation can disrupt the function of electronic devices, even at sea level. Such interactions are rare and unlikely to have a significant effect on the ability of the device to detect and treat life-threatening arrhythmia.

Vibration levels in fixed-wing aircraft are generally low and unlikely to cause problems, except during take off, landing and turbulence when modest increases in pacing rate may occur.

Key points – general management and lifestyle considerations

- General non-pharmacological strategies, including self-care education, treatment adherence, symptom recognition, weight, sodium and fluid management and healthy lifestyle choices are as important as HF-specific medications.
- Patients with HF appear to benefit from exercise as much as others, with a documented improvement in quality of life and a tendency towards reductions in morbidity and mortality.
- Patients with a private driving license are generally restricted from driving only if they have advanced or uncontrolled HF; those with a commercial driving license are banned from driving until further testing.
- Most patients who have had an episode of acute HF should be able to fly, if stable, in 6 weeks. There should be no restriction for patients with chronic HF, although those with NYHA class III or IV should consider airport assistance and request the availability of in-flight oxygen.
- In general, there is no convincing evidence that electromagnetic interference, cosmic radiation or vibration have an important effect on the function of pacemakers or implantable cardiac defibrillators.

Key references

Casas JP, Kwong J, Ebrahim S. Telemonitoring for chronic heart failure: not ready for prime time [editorial]. *Cochrane Database Syst Rev* 2010;8:ED000008.

Clark RA, Inglis SC, McAlister FA et al. Telemonitoring or structured telephone support programmes for patients with chronic heart failure: systematic review and meta-analysis. *BMJ* 2007;334:942.

Dickstein K, Cohen-Solal A, Filippatos G et al. ESC guidelines for the diagnosis and treatment of acute and chronic heart failure 2008. *Eur J Heart Fail* 2008;10:933–89.

Hasan A, Paul V. Telemonitoring in chronic heart failure. *Eur Heart J* 2011;32:1457–64.

Inglis SC, Clark RA, McAlister FA et al. Structured telephone support or telemonitoring programmes for patients with chronic heart failure. *Cochrane Database Syst Rev* 2010;Aug4(8):CD007228.

Krum H, Jelinek MV, Stewart S et al. 2011 update to National Heart Foundation of Australia and Cardiac Society of Australia and New Zealand guidelines for the prevention, detection and management of chronic heart failure in Australia, 2006. *Med J Aust* 2011;194:405–9.

McAlister FA, Stewart S, Ferrua S, Mcmurray JJ. Multidisciplinary strategies for the management of heart failure patients at high risk for admission: a systematic review of randomized trials. *J Am Coll Cardiol* 2004;44:810–19.

Smart N, Marwick TH. Exercise training for patients with heart failure: a systematic review of factors that improve mortality and morbidity. *Am J Med* 2004;116:693–706.

Zografos TA, Katritsis DG. Guidelines and regulations for driving in heart disease. *Hellenic J Cardiol* 2010;51: 226–34.

The different forms of heart failure (HF) (systolic and diastolic, left and right ventricular ([LV/RV] dysfunction, acute and chronic – see Chapter 1) require somewhat different treatment approaches.

While successful evidence-based therapy now exists for HF due to LV systolic dysfunction, the search for the 'holy grail' in diastolic HF (heart failure with preserved ejection fraction [HFpEF]) continues. Several large studies of beta-blockers, angiotensin-converting enzyme (ACE) inhibitors and angiotensin-receptor blockers (ARBs) have not been successful. In general, the management of HFpEF should be directed towards the underlying cause (e.g. lowering blood pressure in patients with hypertension, revascularization in patients with coronary ischemia). Symptoms of congestion should be managed with diuretics (see page 83). Trials of aldosterone antagonists and phosphodiesterase-5 inhibitors in patients with HFpEF are ongoing.

In this chapter, we outline the evidence-based medical therapy for systolic HF.

General management principles

Knowledge of LV and RV function is essential to the application of medical therapy. If LV/RV systolic dysfunction is confirmed, causes should be sought, as ultimately the treatment of HF due to valvular heart disease, myocardial infarction (MI) or severe pulmonary disease will vary because of the different mechanism and ventricle involved. A search for aggravating factors such as drugs (calcium-channel antagonists, namely diltiazem and verapamil; non-steroidal anti-inflammatory drugs [NSAIDs]; cyclooxygenase [COX]-2 inhibitors; class 1 antiarrhythmics; thiazolidinediones) and concomitant problems (arrhythmia, anemia, infection, thromboembolism, thyroid disease) should also be performed and the prescribed therapy modified accordingly.

Monitoring. Successful safe HF therapy requires specific and regular monitoring, including measurement of weight or fluid balance (daily), heart rate, blood pressure (lying and standing), and respiratory rate and oxygen saturation. Regular serum creatinine and electrolyte measurements should be performed according to the clinical scenario, primarily if the patient is on intravenous diuretics, and potassium and magnesium must be replaced if the patient is hypokalemic or hypomagnesemic. Imaging results (chest X-ray and echocardiography) are helpful for assessing the response to treatment.

First-line therapy

Diuretics (in patients with fluid retention/pulmonary congestion) are the oldest agents used in HF therapy. They are very successful in limiting the symptoms of fluid retention but have not been proved to reduce mortality in HF. Symptomatic systolic HF should be treated with a combination of an ACE inhibitor and a diuretic to maintain euvolemia.

Oral diuretics. In mild and stable forms of HF, the oral route should be used first. Loop diuretics and thiazides are prescribed most frequently (Table 7.1). Loop diuretics act on the ascending loop of Henle in the kidney. Dose escalation and addition of a thiazide diuretic may be required if the edema is resistant. However, there is a risk of significant diuresis when a loop diuretic and thiazide are used in combination. Daily weight monitoring and frequent electrolyte measurement should be employed in such cases, with prompt replacement of potassium when required.

Metolazone is a strong diuretic often used in combination with loop diuretics when loop diuretics alone do not work.

Potassium-sparing diuretics are weak diuretics when used alone, and are most frequently used in the treatment of ascites caused by end-stage liver disease. The aldosterone antagonists have an important role in the management of HF (see below).

Acetazolamide is a weak diuretic designed to block tissue carbonic anhydrase. The effect is to lower serum pH, and high dosing may result in metabolic acidosis. The drug is used infrequently, mainly in patients with metabolic alkalosis.

Intravenous diuretics are reserved for patients with acute LV dysfunction or those presenting with edema resistant to oral diuretics. Furosemide can be administered by continuous infusion or boluses. The usual starting dose for intravenous boluses is 40–80 mg at a continuous infusion rate of 5–10 mg/hour. In fluid-overloaded patients, the aim

TABLE 7.1

Examples of oral diuretic treatment for heart failure

	Initial dose
Loop diuretics	
Furosemide	40–80 mg od or bd
Bumetanide	1–2 mg od or bd
Torasemide (torsemide)	10–20 mg od
Thiazides	
Hydrochlorothiazide	25–50 mg od
Bendroflumethiazide	2.5–10 mg od
Quinazolone diuretics	
Metolazone	2.5–5 mg od
Potassium-sparing diuretics	
Amiloride	5–10 mg od
Triamterene	100 mg bd
Aldosterone antagonists (see Table 7.8)	
Other diuretics	
Acetazolamide	250–375 mg od or alternate days

bd, twice daily; od, once daily.

is to achieve an increase in urine output and a weight reduction of 0.5– 1.0 kg/day. Peak diuresis should be achieved within 2 hours and last for 6–8 hours.

General monitoring includes daily weight and serum electrolytes, and large or rapid weight losses should be avoided. The diuretic dose needs to be reassessed regularly and adjusted according to volume status, either by modifying the intravenous dosage or changing to oral therapy.

ACE inhibitors block tissue angiotensin-converting enzyme, which is responsible for the conversion of angiotensin I to angiotensin II, and the breakdown of bradykinin. This causes vasodilation and decreases intraglomerular pressure.

There is strong evidence that ACE inhibitors maximize blockade of the renin–angiotensin–aldosterone system and prevent progression of the disease in all stages of HF with systolic dysfunction (LV ejection fraction [LVEF] < 40%). All patients with systolic LV dysfunction, including asymptomatic patients (NYHA class I) should be treated with ACE inhibitors at target doses (Table 7.2). If target doses are not reached (poorly tolerated), then lower doses are still beneficial. If ACE inhibitors are contraindicated (Table 7.3) or cause specific side effects (cough), then an ARB should be used instead. Absolute and relative contraindications and drug interactions are shown in Table 7.3. There is no convincing evidence for the use of ACE inhibitors in HFpEF.

The CONSENSUS trial was the first study to show prognostic improvement with an ACE inhibitor (enalapril with a target dose of 20 mg twice daily) in patients in NYHA class IV HF. CONSENSUS I reported on survival at 10 years. The results showed that the effect of enalapril was sustained for at least 4 years and mortality was significantly higher in the placebo group.

The SOLVD-T trial randomized 2569 patients already receiving conventional treatment for HF to enalapril, 2.5–20 mg daily, or placebo. There were significant reductions in mortality in the enalapril group (the largest reduction was in those with progressive HF) and fewer patients were hospitalized for worsening HF in this group.

The ATLAS trial was undertaken with the precise objective of comparing two dosages of lisinopril (2.5–5 mg daily and 32.5–35 mg

TABLE 7.2

Examples of ACE inhibitor treatment for heart failure

	Starting dose	Target dose
Enalapril	2.5 mg bd	20 mg bd
Lisinopril	2.5–5 mg od	20–35 mg od
Ramipril	1.25 mg bd	5 mg bd
Trandolapril	0.5 mg od	4 mg od
Captopril	6.25 mg tds	50 mg tds
Perindopril	2.5 mg od	10 mg od

ACE, angiotensin-converting enzyme; bd, twice daily; od, once daily; tds, three times daily.

TABLE 7.3

Contraindications and drug interactions of ACE inhibitors

Absolute contraindications	Relative contraindications	Drug interactions
History of anaphylaxis	Significant hyperkalemia (> 5.0 mmol/L)	K+ supplements or K+-sparing diuretics (e.g. triamterene)
Angioneurotic edema	Significant renal dysfunction (eGFR < 30 mL/min)	Aldosterone antagonists (spironolactone)
Known bilateral renal artery stenosis	Symptomatic or severe asymptomatic hypotension (systolic BP < 90 mmHg)	ARBs
Acute kidney failure	Hyponatremia with volume depletion	NSAIDs

ACE, angiotensin-converting enzyme; ARB, angiotensin-receptor blocker; BP, blood pressure; eGFR, estimated glomerular filtration rate; NSAID, non-steroidal anti-inflammatory drug.

daily) on the morbidity and mortality of patients with LV systolic dysfunction. 3000 patients with NYHA class II–IV were followed up for 4.5 years. The high-dose group had a significant 12% lower risk of death or hospitalization for any reason, and 24% fewer cases of hospitalization for HF.

Other trials. SAVE, AIRE and TRACE have all clearly demonstrated the benefits of ACE inhibitors in reducing mortality and morbidity in patients with systolic HF after MI.

Angiotensin-receptor blockers are first-line treatments in patients with NYHA class II–IV HF who are intolerant to an ACE inhibitor, and second-line treatment after optimal ACE inhibitor and beta-blocker therapy in patients with NYHA class III or IV (Table 7.4). Absolute and relative contraindications and drug interactions are shown in Table 7.5.

The Val-HEFT trial randomized 5010 patients with NYHA class II–IV to valsartan, 40 mg twice daily titrated to 160 mg twice daily, or placebo.

TABLE 7.4

Examples of ARB treatment for heart failure

	Starting dose	Target dose
Candesartan	4 or 8 mg od	16 mg bd
Valsartan	40 mg bd	160 mg bd
Irbesartan	75 mg od	300 mg od

ARB, angiotensin-receptor blocker; bd, twice daily; od, once daily.

TABLE 7.5

Contraindications and drug interactions for angiotensin receptor blockers

Absolute contraindications	Relative contraindications	Drug interactions
Acute/severe renal failure	Significant hyperkalemia (> 5.0 mmol/L)	K+ supplements or K+-sparing diuretics (e.g. triamterene)
Acute/severe liver failure	Symptomatic or severe asymptomatic hypotension (systolic BP < 90 mmHg)	Aldosterone antagonists (spironolactone, eplerenone); ACE inhibitors; NSAIDs

ACE, angiotensin-converting enzyme; BP; blood pressure; NSAID, non-steroidal anti-inflammatory drug.

Mean follow-up was 23 months. The valsartan group demonstrated a significantly reduced combined HF mortality and morbidity of 13.2%, and reduced hospitalization for HF by 27.5%.

The CHARM trial randomized 4576 patients to candesartan or placebo in two complementary parallel trials: CHARM-Alternative with patients who could not tolerate ACE inhibitors and CHARM-Added with patients who were already receiving ACE inhibitors. In both groups, candesartan significantly reduced all-cause mortality, cardiovascular death and HF hospitalizations.

The **VALIANT** *trial* enrolled 14 703 patients into three treatment arms: valsartan titrated to 160 mg twice daily; captopril titrated to 50 mg three times daily; and valsartan, 80 mg twice daily, plus captopril, 50 mg three times daily. Patients had HF and/or LV dysfunction after acute MI. The results showed that valsartan was as effective as captopril but combining valsartan with captopril increased the rate of adverse events.

Beta-blockers. Over the past 25 years, a large number of trials have investigated the effects of beta-blockade in patients with HF and provided clear evidence supporting their use in the context of HF with significant systolic dysfunction. As a result, beta-blockers have become a part of contemporary therapy alongside ACE inhibitors and diuretics. All patients with stable HF (NYHA class II or III) are suitable candidates for beta-blocker treatment after euvolemia is achieved. In patients with severe HF (NYHA class IV), beta-blockers should be initiated under close supervision, preferably in a hospital setting. In general, to minimize the small risk of precipitating HF, beta-blockers should be commenced at low doses and uptitrated (every 2 weeks) while ensuring the patient's clinical status remains stable. If target doses are not tolerated, then lower doses are still beneficial (Table 7.6). Contraindications and drug interactions are shown in Table 7.7.

Randomized clinical trials of beta-blocker therapy in HF confirm the substantial clinical benefits to be gained with this therapy; other trials have added further understanding of the potential modes of action underlying these clinical effects such as anti-ischemic and anti-LV remodeling.

TABLE 7.6

Examples of beta-blocker treatment for heart failure

	Starting dose	Target dose
Carvedilol	3.125 mg bd	25–50 mg bd
Metoprolol CR/XL	23.75 mg od	190 mg od
Bisoprolol	1.25 mg od	10 mg od
Nebivolol	1.25 mg od	10 mg od

bd, twice daily; od, once daily.

TABLE 7.7

Contraindications and drug interactions of beta-blockers

Absolute contraindications	Relative contraindications	Drug interactions
Acute LV failure	Asthma	Digoxin
AV conduction disease	Bradycardia (HR < 60 bpm), and hypotension (systolic BP < 90 mmHg)	Amiodarone
Sinus bradycardia < 50 bpm	Persisting signs of congestion, peripheral edema/ascites	

AV, atrioventricular; BP, blood pressure; bpm, beats per minute; HR, heart rate; LV, left ventricular; RV, right ventricular.

The CIBIS II trial randomized 2647 HF patients (NYHA class III or IV) to placebo or bisoprolol (titrated to 10 mg daily). The trial was stopped early as bisoprolol showed significant mortality benefit. All-cause mortality was lower in the bisoprolol group than those on placebo (11.8% vs 17.3%).

The MERIT-HF trial enrolled 3991 patients with NYHA class II–IV stabilized on standard therapy, of whom 1990 patients were randomized to metoprolol succinate (extended release) and 2001 patients were assigned to placebo. This study was also stopped early as all-cause mortality was lower in the metoprolol group than the placebo group (7.2% vs 11%).

The COMET trial randomized 3029 patients (NYHA class II–IV) to carvedilol (target dose 25 mg twice daily) or metoprolol tartrate (target dose 50 mg twice daily). Although the mortality result clearly favored carvedilol (17% relative risk reduction), an immediate-release formulation of metoprolol was used, which was different from the formulation used in the MERIT-HF trial (see above).

The CAPRICORN trial enrolled 1959 patients who had had an acute MI with LV dysfunction. These patients were treated with carvedilol (target dose 25 mg twice daily). A 23% reduction in the primary endpoint of all-cause mortality was reported.

The COPERNICUS trial randomized 2289 patients with severe (NYHA class IV) HF to carvedilol (target dose 25 mg twice daily) or placebo. The trial was stopped early after 10.4 months because of the highly significant beneficial effect of carvedilol on survival. Mortality was reduced by 34% in the treatment group, with carvedilol also reducing the number of days spent in hospital for HF by 40%.

The SENIORS trial was the first HF trial restricted to an elderly population (mean age of 76) and included patients who had relative preservation of LV systolic function. A total of 2128 patients were randomized to nebivolol (target dose 10 mg) or placebo. The primary composite endpoint of all-cause mortality or hospital admissions for cardiovascular events was significantly reduced by 14% in the treatment group.

Heart failure with normal systolic function. Despite the compelling evidence that beta-blockers improve the prognosis of systolic HF there are limited data regarding the role of beta-blockers in HF with normal systolic function (diastolic dysfunction). The introduction of beta-blockers with vasodilating properties (nebivolol, carvedilol) has renewed interest in this area. Large-scale long-term clinical trials are required to address the long-term effects of beta-blockers on clinical status and prognosis in this patient group.

Systolic heart failure and diabetes mellitus. Historically, the use of beta-blockers in patients with diabetes has been questioned in view of the potential negative effect on insulin sensitivity and risk of more severe hypoglycemic attacks. In trials, treatment with carvedilol has been associated with an improvement in clinical symptoms, LV function, and resting and exercise hemodynamic variables, with no significant difference between patients with and without diabetes. The incidence of adverse effects appeared to be similar in the two groups. Other analyses with the selective beta-blockers bisoprolol and metoprolol suggest similar results for patients with and without diabetes. As expected, patients with diabetes had higher all-cause mortality than patients without diabetes.

Systolic heart failure and chronic obstructive pulmonary disease (COPD). The beneficial effect of beta blockade in this group is difficult to ascertain as such patients have been excluded from large randomized trials. However, long-term beta-blocker therapy after MI has been shown to improve survival in patients with and without COPD. Until recently, beta-blockers have been generally avoided in patients with COPD for fear of inducing bronchospasm. Several small studies and a subsequent meta-analysis have suggested a good safety record with low to moderate doses of selective beta-1-receptor blockers in this clinical setting. However, dose escalation leads to loss of selectivity and a potential risk of bronchospasm. A meta-analysis of randomized placebo-controlled trials of selective beta-blockers in reactive airways disease has supported the lack of significant effects on forced expiration volume in 1 second (FEV_1), bronchodilator response to beta-2-receptor stimulation and symptoms.

Carvedilol, with its combination of non-selective beta- and alpha-adrenergic blockade has also been safely used in patients with COPD and HF.

Despite limited trial data and clinical experience, patients with HF and COPD with no history of long-standing wheezing and/or no evidence of reversible airways obstruction on objective testing should not be denied the substantial benefit of beta-blockers. In many cases an informed choice by the patient, with full understanding of the risks and potential benefits of these agents, is required. As a rule, however, the dose in these patients should be carefully titrated and high doses generally avoided. As there are no safety data for beta-blockers in patients presenting with acute exacerbations of COPD, the use of these agents in this setting should be avoided.

Systolic heart failure and end-stage renal disease. Patients with end-stage renal disease and evidence of systolic HF have been reported to have a 2-year mortality in excess of 70%. Selective beta-blockers (including metoprolol) have shown rather unfavorable effects on renal hemodynamics, with concomitant falls in systemic blood pressure and renal blood flow and an increase in renal vascular resistance. In contrast, carvedilol does not change renal blood flow despite a fall in systemic blood pressure, decreases renal vascular resistance because of its prominent vasodilatory properties and does not require dose adjustment as it is primarily metabolized by the liver.

Systolic left-sided heart failure in the elderly. HF is predominantly a disease of the elderly, with 50% of HF in patients aged over 75 years. Overall, the survival benefit from beta-blockers in elderly patients with HF (including nebivolol) is modest and a proportion of elderly patients will experience adverse effects.

For elderly patients with systolic left-sided HF, the adverse effects of beta-blocker treatment on quality of life need to be balanced against the likely mortality benefits. For those individuals who can tolerate a beta-blocker, judicious use of the drug is likely to be beneficial. Titration of beta-blocker doses should be guided by the patient's symptoms, with recognition that elderly patients are less likely to achieve maximum doses and more likely to experience adverse effects.

Aldosterone antagonists block the action of aldosterone at the mineralocorticoid receptors within the heart that mediate fibrosis, hypertrophy and arrhythmogenesis. These agents should be considered in patients who remain symptomatic (NYHA class II–IV) despite appropriate doses of ACE inhibitors and beta-blockers. A 'selective' aldosterone antagonist without an anti-androgenic effect, eplerenone, has been found to reduce mortality and hospitalization after MI, in patients with reduced LV systolic function and symptoms of HF. Thus, eplerenone should be considered within 2 weeks of MI in patients with an LVEF below 40% (Table 7.8).

Before treatment, baseline serum potassium should be less than 5.0 mmol/L and estimated glomerular filtration rate (eGFR) should be greater than 30 mL/minute. Aldosterone antagonists should be initiated at a low dose and then uptitrated while checking tolerance and blood chemistry (potassium). Contraindications and drug interactions are shown in Table 7.9.

RALES trial randomized 1663 patients with severe HF, who were already receiving an ACE inhibitor, loop diuretic and in most cases digoxin, to spironolactone, 25 mg, or placebo. The trial was discontinued

TABLE 7.8

Examples of aldosterone antagonist treatment for heart failure

	Starting dose	Target dose
Spironolactone	12.5 mg od (if GFR > 30 and < 49 mL/min)	50 mg od
	25 mg od (if GFR > 50 mL/min)	
Canrenone	50 mg od	200 mg daily
Eplerenone	25 mg od	50 mg od

GFR, glomerular filtration rate; od, once daily.

TABLE 7.9

Contraindications and drug interactions of aldosterone antagonists

Absolute contraindications	Relative contraindications	Drug interactions
Severe hyperkalemia	Significant hyperkalemia (> 5.0 mmol/L)	K^+ supplements or K^+-sparing diuretics (e.g. triamterene)
Acute renal failure	Significant renal dysfunction	ACE inhibitors; ARBs; NSAIDs

ACE, angiotensin-converting enzyme; ARB, angiotensin-receptor blocker; NSAID, non-steroidal anti-inflammatory drug.

early after 24 months as the spironolactone group showed significant reduction in mortality and rate of hospitalization, and improvement in HF symptoms.

EPHESUS trial enrolled 6642 patients who had had an MI within the previous 3–14 days. They were randomized to eplerenone, 25 mg daily (target dose 50 mg daily) or placebo. In the eplerenone group there was a significant 15% reduction in total all-cause mortality and 13% fewer cardiovascular-related deaths or hospitalizations than in the placebo group.

EMPHASIS trial enrolled 2737 patients with mild HF symptoms (including NYHA class II) to receive eplerenone, 25 mg daily (target dose 50 mg daily) or placebo. The trial was stopped prematurely at 21 months as significant benefits were found in the eplerenone group compared with placebo: a 24% reduction in the rate of death from any cause and a 42% reduction in the rate of hospitalization for HF.

Second-line therapy

Heart rate reduction. Patients with cardiac disease and baseline heart rates greater than or equal to 70 beats per minute have a significantly greater risk of all-cause and cardiovascular mortality, as well as a higher risk of HF hospitalizations.

Ivabradine is a selective inhibitor of a sodium–potassium channel highly expressed in the sinoatrial node. Its pharmacological actions lead to

93

a slowing of the heart rate in patients with preserved sinus rhythm. A recent large randomized controlled study (SHIFT) in patients with symptomatic HF with recent hospitalization (LVEF < 35%, heart rate > 70 beats per minute [bpm]) found that ivabradine reduced mortality from HF and hospitalization for worsening HF. Patients on active treatment were found to have less cardiac remodeling and improved LVEF. However, only 25% of patients reached the target beta-blocker dose.

The drug can be used when the heart rate remains elevated (> 70 bpm) after beta-blocker titration, where beta-blockers are contraindicated (e.g. in severe bronchial asthma) or poorly tolerated. Ivabradine is not available in the USA.

Omega-3 polyunsaturated fatty acids have been shown to reduce mortality and HF rehospitalization rate compared with placebo (GISSI-HF trial). Polyunsaturated fatty acids should be considered for patients who remain symptomatic despite standard therapy. A dose of 1 g daily of almost pure omega-3 polyunsaturated fatty acid or equivalent is recommended.

Digoxin may be considered for symptom relief and to reduce the need for hospitalization in patients who are already on first-line therapy. It also remains a valuable therapy for patients with atrial fibrillation (AF). Check serum levels: the recommended therapeutic level is 0.5–0.8 ng/mL for HF. Beware of drug toxicity, mainly in patients with renal dysfunction. Common side effects include nausea and anorexia; these can develop even if the serum level is within the therapeutic range. Caution should be taken when increasing beta-blocker dosage, as the digoxin dose may need to be reduced or stopped.

Nitrates and hydralazine may be considered in patients who are intolerant of, or have contraindications to, ACE inhibitors and ARBs.

Other therapies
Anticoagulation is advised in patients with LV dysfunction and AF/atrial flutter, intracardiac thrombus or LV aneurysm. It can also be considered for patients with severe systolic LV dysfunction. Choice of agents includes warfarin, dabigatran (a novel direct thrombin inhibitor) or factor Xa inhibitors rivaroxaban and apixaban (where approved). Unless

contraindicated, prophylaxis for deep vein thrombosis should be administered to patients with severe HF who are slow to mobilize.

Intravenous iron replacement should be considered in iron-deficient anemic patients, while patients with severe obstructive sleep apnea can be treated with nasal continuous positive airway pressure (if tolerated) (see Chapter 4).

Potentially harmful drugs to avoid in patients with HF are listed in Table 7.10.

Inotropic agents

Intravenous inotropic agents (drugs that increase the strength of heart muscle contraction) such as dopamine, dobutamine and milrinone are used in patients with acute decompensated HF, as they stabilize cardiac output and blood pressure and support adequate blood supply to vital organs (kidneys, heart) until more definitive therapy is introduced (e.g. revascularization, LV assist device).

TABLE 7.10

Potentially harmful drugs to avoid in heart failure

- NSAIDs and COX-2 inhibitors increase the risk of fluid retention and renal failure
- Non-dihydropyridine calcium-channel blockers with negative inotropic effect (diltiazem and verapamil), moxonidine, clozapine and glitazones
- TCAs and SNRIs (venlafaxine, reboxetine)
- Corticosteroids

Consider the potential effects of the following.

- Effervescent products (e.g. Ural sachets, Panadol soluble, Aspro Clear, Eno)[*] on serum potassium levels in patients receiving ACE inhibitor/ARB/aldosterone antagonist treatment
- Fiber supplements (e.g. Metamucil, Fybogel)[*] on daily fluid intake, as they need a large amount of fluid to work.

[*]Brand names vary in different countries.
ACE, angiotensin-converting enzyme; ARB, angiotensin-receptor blocker; COX, cyclooxygenase; NSAID, non-steroidal anti-inflammatory drug; SNRI, serotonin and norepinephrine reuptake inhibitor; TCA, tricyclic antidepressant.

Long-term use of moderate to high doses of inotropic agents is associated with excessive mortality (due to the increase in oxygen debt of the working myocardium) and should be avoided. The effects of low-dose or intermittent infusion are not yet known; the results of a study of low-dose dopamine infusion (< 5 µg/kg/minute) in patients with cardiorenal syndrome are awaited.

Some HF centers use intravenous inotropic agents in ambulatory patients with severe intractable HF ('pulsed therapy'). Although this intermittent therapy provides some patients with hemodynamic and clinical improvement, the potential for life-threatening arrhythmia and rebound HF in between treatments is a concern.

Newer agents (calcium sensitizers) have shown initial promise but so far have not demonstrated a significant advantage in terms of mortality over inotropes.

Treatment of acute heart failure

Patients with acute HF require prompt clinical assessment and initial medical stabilization tailored to the underlying problem before a smooth transition to the chronic HF management phase. The therapeutic target – cardiac output, blood pressure or intravascular volume – should dictate the initial intervention (Table 7.11).

Patients with known LV dysfunction who present with acute HF will already be receiving HF medication. On admission, oral diuretics are usually changed to intravenous loop diuretics, while vasodilators (ACE inhibitors, ARBs) are continued. Aldosterone antagonists should be stopped in patients with progressive renal dysfunction, and ACE inhibitor/ ARB therapy reviewed. Beta-blockers are only withheld in acute pulmonary edema or incipient cardiogenic shock. Otherwise, beta-blocker therapy should continue. Use of beta-blockers in patients receiving inotropic support (e.g. dopamine and dobutamine) appears to be counterproductive.

Importantly, heparin prophylaxis for deep vein thrombosis should be used in all patients with acute HF (unless contraindicated).

TABLE 7.11

Treatment of acute heart failure

Clinical findings	Treatment
Normal or moderately raised BP and pulmonary congestion	Initial i.v. diuretic therapy ± vasodilators
High BP	Initial i.v. vasodilators ± diuretics
Flash pulmonary edema	i.v. vasodilators, i.v. diuretics and non-invasive ventilation
Low systolic BP (< 100 mmHg) but no evidence of cardiogenic shock	Initial inotropic agents with vasodilator properties (dobutamine, milrinone, levosimendan) and digoxin
Cardiogenic shock	Vasopressors (dopamine, noradrenaline)
	Consider invasive mechanical support (intra-aortic balloon pump, LVAD) before revascularization or transplant
Pulmonary embolism	Assess for surgery (embolectomy) or lysis
Acute MI	Lysis and angioplasty
RV dysfunction	
• due to severe pulmonary arterial hypertension	Pulmonary vasodilators
• due to acute MI	Maintain preload and revascularization
Recovering from cardiac surgery	Initial diuretic therapy
	Search for precipitant (arrhythmia, ischemia, ongoing LV remodeling, new RV dysfunction, excessive perioperative volume) and treat accordingly

BP, blood pressure; i.v., intravenous; LV, left ventricular; LVAD, left ventricular assist device; MI, myocardial infarction; RV, right ventricular.

Key points – pharmacological management

- Medical management of heart failure (HF) with preserved systolic function remains challenging, but in principle should target the underlying cause (e.g. blood pressure, coronary ischemia).
- Diuretics, angiotensin-converting enzyme (ACE) inhibitors, angiotensin-receptor blockers (ARBs), beta-blockers and aldosterone antagonists are the mainstay of therapy for symptomatic left ventricular systolic dysfunction.
- Second-line agents: digoxin, ivabradine, omega-3 polyunsaturated fatty acids and vasodilators (nitrates and hydralazine) should be considered in particular clinical scenarios (ongoing symptoms with recurrent admissions to hospital, excessive heart rate in sinus rhythm or atrial fibrillation and contraindications to ACE inhibitors and ARBs).
- Inotropic agents are used short term in acute cases with severe cardiac dysfunction (cardiogenic shock) and can be supplemented by mechanical circulatory support (e.g. intra-aortic balloon pump, left ventricular assist device).
- Acute HF is a medical emergency and the treatment has to be tailored to the underlying clinical problem (lowering blood pressure in severe hypertension, revascularization in acute myocardial infarction).

Key references

CIBIS-II. The Cardiac Insufficiency Bisoprolol Study II (CIBIS-II): a randomised trial. *Lancet* 1999;353: 9–13.

The CONSENSUS Trial Study Group. Effects of enalapril on mortality in severe congestive heart failure: results of the Cooperative North Scandinavian Enalapril Survival Study (CONSENSUS). *N Engl J Med* 1987;316:1429–35.

Flather MD, Shibata MC, Coats AJ et al. Randomized trial to determine the effect of nebivolol on mortality and cardiovascular hospital admission in elderly patients with heart failure (SENIORS). *Eur Heart J* 2005;26: 215–25.

Gheorghiade M, Pang PS. Acute heart failure syndromes. *J Am Coll Cardiol* 2009;53:557–73.

Granger CB, Mcmurray JJ, Yusuf S et al. Effects of candesartan in patients with chronic heart failure and reduced left-ventricular systolic function intolerant to angiotensin-converting-enzyme inhibitors: the CHARM-Alternative trial. *Lancet* 2003;362:772–6.

McMurray J, Cohen-Solal A, Dietz R et al. Practical recommendations for the use of ACE inhibitors, beta-blockers, aldosterone antagonists and angiotensin receptor blockers in heart failure: putting guidelines into practice. *Eur J Heart Fail* 2005;7:710–21.

MERIT-HF. Effect of metoprolol CR/XL in chronic heart failure: Metoprolol CR/XL Randomised Intervention Trial in Congestive Heart Failure (MERIT-HF). *Lancet* 1999;353:2001–7.

Packer M, Coats AJ, Fowler MB et al. Effect of carvedilol on survival in severe chronic heart failure. *N Engl J Med* 2001;344:1651–8.

Packer M, Poole-Wilson PA, Armstrong PW et al. Comparative effects of low and high doses of the angiotensin-converting enzyme inhibitor, lisinopril, on morbidity and mortality in chronic heart failure. *Circulation* 1999;100:2312–18.

Pitt B, Zannad F, Remme WJ et al. The effect of spironolactone on morbidity and mortality in patients with severe heart failure. Randomized Aldactone Evaluation Study Investigators. *N Engl J Med* 1999;341:709–17.

Implantable cardiac defibrillators

Death from heart failure (HF) is usually related to pump failure or, if sudden, ventricular arrhythmia (Figure 8.1). Left ventricular ejection fraction (LVEF) tends to be a predictor of outcome and sudden death. The majority of clinical trials have shown an increased risk of ventricular arrhythmias when LVEF is reduced to 30–35% or lower. A number of clinical trials have shown a mortality benefit in patients receiving an implantable cardiac defibrillator (ICD) either as primary or secondary prevention (Table 8.1).

Approximately 10% of patients who have an ICD for primary prevention receive an appropriate shock in the first 2 years after the device is implanted. Patients who receive an ICD for secondary prevention have a high risk of recurrence without treatment, with a rate of sudden death of up to 40% 1 year after presentation. Pharmacological therapy (e.g. amiodarone) is not effective at preventing sudden death and an ICD is superior therapy.

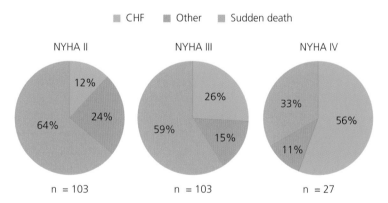

Figure 8.1 Data from the MERIT-HF trial show that the risk of sudden death is greatest when patients are NYHA class II and that death from pump failure is greater in advanced symptomatic heart failure (NYHA class IV).
CHF, chronic heart failure; NYHA, New York Heart Association. Source: *Lancet* 1999;353:2001–7, reproduced with permission from Elsevier © 1999.

TABLE 8.1

Recommendations for ICD implantation*

Primary prevention

- LV dysfunction (LVEF ≤ 35%), prior MI/IHD and at least 40 days post acute MI
- LV dysfunction (LVEF ≤ 35%) of non-ischemic etiology
- High risk of SCD (e.g. familial long QT, some cases of hypertrophic myopathy)

Secondary prevention

- Survivor of cardiac arrest due to VF/VT, after excluding reversible cause
- Structural heart disease with sustained VT
- Syncope, LVEF ≤ 35% and inducible sustained VT/VF at electrophysiological study

*Assuming patient has an overall life expectancy > 1 year, with good functional status.

ICD, implantable cardiac defibrillator; IHD, ischemic heart disease; LV, left ventricular; LVEF, left ventricular ejection fraction; MI, myocardial infarction; SCD, sudden cardiac death; VF, ventricular fibrillation; VT, ventricular tachycardia.

ICDs are usually implanted in the left prepectoral area (they can, if required, be implanted on the right) and are inserted under conscious sedation. The battery life of a modern device is about 5–10 years. The complications are similar to those experienced with pacemakers (see *Fast Facts: Cardiac Arrhythmias*).

Cardiac resynchronization therapy

Hypertension, myocardial infarction (MI) and ischemia can all cause myocardial cell damage and areas of fibrosis. Fibrosis can damage the conduction system of the heart, thereby slowing impulses and promoting cell-to-cell conduction, which is a much slower depolarizing process. This results in a broadening of the QRS complex, often with left bundle branch block type morphology. In many cases there is a differential effect in the contractile function of the ventricles known as ventricular dyssynchrony, in which parts of the ventricle no longer achieve maximum contractility and move at different rates and with a different contractile force to other parts. There are two types of ventricular dyssynchrony:

- intraventricular dyssynchrony, in which the muscle fibers within the left ventricle contract at differing rates and speeds
- interventricular dyssynchrony in which the left and right ventricles no longer contract simultaneously.

Dyssynchrony results in a loss of efficient ventricular contraction and impairs stroke volume and cardiac output. Often there is also dyssynchrony of contraction of the papillary muscles that control mitral valve function, resulting in mitral valve regurgitation which further impairs cardiac output (see pages 26–7).

To improve overall cardiac function the right and left ventricles need to be paced simultaneously. Right ventricular (RV) pacing is a well-established, safe and effective technology. Placing a pacing lead within the left ventricular (LV) cavity is also feasible, but it is fraught with potential problems, particularly thromboembolism to the systemic circulation. Instead, a pacing lead is placed into the coronary sinus, which runs under the heart between the left atrium and ventricle, and then into the peripheral veins under the left ventricle so that the myocardium can be paced reliably. Accessing these veins has been a technical challenge but with better delivery tools the success rate of placing a lead in a satisfactory position is now high.

The technology. In patients with sinus rhythm, three pacing leads are inserted: one to the right atrium, one to the right ventricle (usually at the apex) and one within the coronary sinus to access a posterolateral vein underneath the left ventricle (Figure 8.2). (In patients with atrial fibrillation there is no requirement for an atrial lead.) The coronary sinus ostium is accessed using a specialized sheath system. Once the sheath is placed within the body of the sinus a balloon occlusive catheter is inserted. The balloon is expanded to occlude the vein and contrast is injected through the catheter and a venogram taken (Figure 8.3). This allows the anatomic details of the side veins of the coronary sinus to be documented (see Figure 8.3). A pacing lead and guide wire are then inserted into the sheath and the lead is advanced over the wire into its final position (Figure 8.4).

The leads are connected to a pacing generator. During sinus rhythm, the device senses the underlying p wave and via a short atrioventricular (AV) delay (this must be shorter than intrinsic AV nodal conduction)

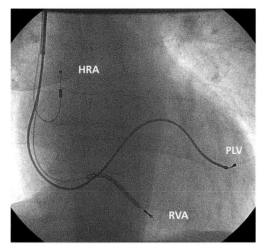

Figure 8.2 Cardiac resynchronization therapy. An anterior–posterior chest X-ray showing the final lead positions: a pacing lead to the high right atrium (HRA), a defibrillating lead at the right ventricular apex (RVA) and a pacing lead within the posterolateral coronary sinus vein (PLV).

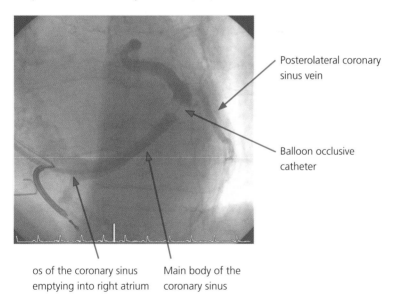

Figure 8.3 Venogram showing the positioning of a balloon occlusive catheter in the coronary sinus and the location of the posterolateral coronary side vein.

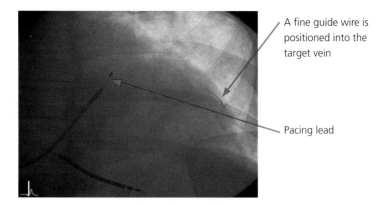

A fine guide wire is positioned into the target vein

Pacing lead

Figure 8.4 Chest X-ray showing the position of the pacing lead within a sheath, which slides over the guide wire. Once the lead in is position and stable the sheath is removed by cutting it away from the lead.

'force' paces the ventricles. The ventricles are continuously driven or paced by the device and intrinsic conduction is suppressed.

Types of device. The basic requirement for cardiac resynchronization therapy (CRT) is to be able to pace both ventricles simultaneously. It is recommended that the device should pace the ventricles at least 92% of the time to exert its full benefit. A device may be either a pacemaker (CRT-P) or a pacemaker and defibrillator (CRT-D), but there is some controversy about which device is best. Patients with less symptomatic HF (NYHA class II or III) are at relatively greater risk of sudden death, whereas patients with ambulatory class IV are more likely to suffer pump failure. There is therefore an argument to implant a CRT-D in patients with fewer symptoms and a CRT-P in those with advanced symptoms.

The CARE-HF study showed that most of the survival benefit of the device was related to CRT-P, while the COMPANION study showed no significant difference between CRT-P and CRT-D in terms of reduction in sudden deaths. Although there are no convincing data of a significant benefit of CRT-D, in the real world a CRT-D device is usually implanted because all patients will have impaired LV function.

Cost implications. CRT is considerably more expensive than standard pacing, often three to four times the cost, and there is a significant cost difference between the CRT-P (AUS$15 000) and CRT-D (AUS$35 000) devices (see above). As the incidence of HF increases, there will be a need for more implants, substantially increasing the cost to society.

Does CRT reduce mortality? The landmark CARE-HF trial studied 813 patients with symptomatic NYHA class II or III HF despite optimal medical treatment; 50% were randomized to continue optimal medical treatment with ACE inhibitors/beta-blockers and diuretics, and 50% additionally underwent implantation of a CRT pacemaker. Mortality was reduced by 32% in the CRT group (Figure 8.5). The readmission rate with decompensated HF was also significantly reduced, as were sudden deaths and overall mortality. As a result, CRT is now standard therapy for patients with HF, broad QRS complexes and symptoms despite optimal medical treatment (Table 8.2).

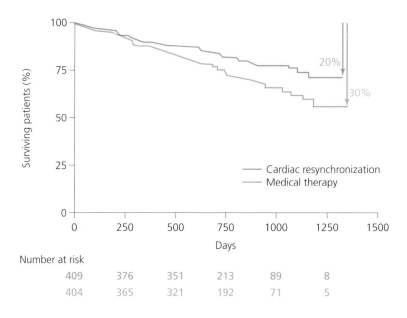

Number at risk

409	376	351	213	89	8
404	365	321	192	71	5

Figure 8.5 The results of the CARE-HF study show a significant mortality reduction (P<0.002) in HF patients implanted with a CRT pacemaker compared with those who received optimal pharmacological treatment only (see text). Adapted from Cleland JGF et al. *N Engl J Med* 2005;352:1539–49.

TABLE 8.2

Inclusion criteria for cardiac resynchronization therapy

- Impaired LV function: LVEF < 35%
- NYHA class III and ambulatory class IV symptoms of HF despite optimal medical treatment with ACE inhibitors or ARBs/beta-blockers/diuretics and spironolactone
- Wide QRS complexes > 120 ms, preferably with a LBBB morphology
- Reasonable expectation of life > 1 year
- Sinus rhythm or atrial fibrillation*
- CRT-D (defibrillation) or CRT-P (pacemaker) depends on clinical judgment

*CRT for patients with atrial fibrillation, providing pacing occurs for more than 92% of the time. If not, consider atrioventricular nodal ablation.
ACE, angiotensin-converting enzyme; ARB, angiotensin-receptor blocker; HF heart failure; LBBB, left bundle branch block; LVEF, left ventricular ejection fraction; NYHA, New York Heart Association.

Does CRT improve morbidity? Many studies have consistently shown an improvement in NYHA symptoms, usually decreasing by at least one class, sometimes two or even three. These changes are maintained for at least 2 years and there is evidence that the improvements occur over the duration of the device. Exercise capacity is significantly increased, as is quality of life. There is also a significant reduction in the readmission rate for decompensated HF. There is also some evidence that CRT slows down the progression of HF.

Does everyone benefit? Virtually all studies have shown that 20–30% of patients fail to demonstrate a positive outcome ('non-responders'). Failure is defined as little change in symptoms or outcome, but in many studies the definition of failure is controversial. As these devices are expensive, identifying patients who may not benefit is critically important. There are a number of factors which make the device less likely to be beneficial but none of these is currently felt to be absolute. Cardiac MRI can show a full-thickness posterior MI, and has been used to decide if placing a lead in the posterior coronary sinus veins is worthwhile; often it is not. Echocardiography has been used to look at a number of variables of dyssynchrony but there has been a lack of reproducibility.

Possible contraindications are shown in Table 8.3. Cost-effectiveness for ICDs is significantly reduced in patients over 75–80 years of age (Figure 8.6), and clinical judgment should be used in very elderly patients. Although patients with mild (NYHA class I) symptoms do not appear to benefit, recent trials (Reverse and MADIT-CRT) suggest that early implantation of the device slows down the progression of HF and allows positive LV remodeling. Increasingly, CRT is used earlier in treatment.

Patients with systolic HF and a QRS greater than 120 ms with optimal medical treatment should be referred for assessment.

Although non-responders are a significant issue, some patients respond very significantly ('super-responders'). Identifying these patients has also been a challenge. Often the only way to know for sure whether the patient will respond is to implant the device.

Do these systems need regular maintenance? All devices need to be interrogated on a regular basis throughout their life, usually every 6 months to test lead integrity and battery life. In addition, for CRT patients in sinus rhythm these devices can be 'optimized' to provide the best hemodynamic response. Some modern devices are capable of automatic optimization, which can be carried out at regular intervals, but otherwise it is a time-consuming intervention. Each patient must be

TABLE 8.3

Possible contraindications for CRT device implantation

- Poor ventricular rate control in atrial fibrillation (AV nodal ablation is recommended to ensure pacing is constant)
- Right bundle branch block
- Full-thickness posterior MI (can affect lead positioning)
- Narrow QRS complexes (< 120 ms)
- Mild symptoms

AV, atrioventricular; CRT, cardiac resynchronization therapy; MI, myocardial infarction.

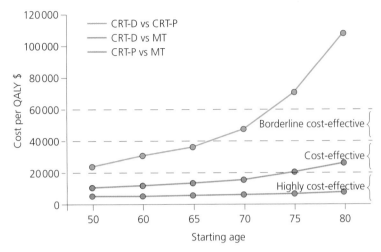

Figure 8.6 Comparison of the cost-effectiveness of a CRT pacemaker (CRT-P) versus a CRT combined pacemaker and defibrillator (CRT-D), and each device compared with medical treatment. Both devices (CRT-P and CRT-D) are cost-effective compared with medical treatment only in patients under 75 years old. CRT, cardiac resynchronization therapy; MT, medical treatment; QALY, quality-adjusted life-year.

individualized and often more than once, perhaps twice per year. In addition, optimization may be needed during exercise.

Is implantation safe? Current systems are safe to implant, with overall mortality less than 0.5%. Specific risks relating to CRT include:
• failure to implant the left ventricular leads
• late lead displacement (8%)
• phrenic nerve stimulation (10%).
  Other risks are similar to those of any standard pacemaker implant:
• pneumothorax (1%)
• infection (early < 1%; late 1.5%)
• lead dislodgement (1–5%).

Cardiac surgery
The aim of specific surgery for HF over and above valve replacement and coronary bypass is to reduce the LV size and volume, and remove 'redundant' or scar tissue (surgical ventricular restoration, variants are

known eponymously as the Batista and Dor procedures). The STICH trial compared routine bypass surgery in patients with impaired LV function with an additional procedure to reduce LV volume in patients with large anterior wall scars. The outcomes were similar in both groups; the reduction in LV volumes did not confer an outcome advantage. Thus, reductive LV surgery should only be considered in patients with severe LV dilatation and HF but needs to be individualized and balanced against the risks.

Mitral valve surgery is covered in Chapters 3 and 10.

Left ventricle assist device. Although contemporary medical therapy with vasodilators, beta-blockers and aldosterone antagonists (see Chapter 7) provides a significant impact on the mortality and morbidity of advanced HF, it is not sufficient in patients with severe symptoms. Cardiac transplantation in this setting is very effective, with 10-year survival rates approaching 50%, but in view of the shortage of organs it remains trivial. Mechanical pumps that take over the function of the damaged ventricle have therefore been developed to stabilize the patient's condition when hemodynamic compromise ensues, either as a result of acute illness (MI, myocarditis, postpartum) or in the process of ongoing LV remodeling (in chronic HF). These devices unload the damaged ventricle (mainly LV) either by redirecting the blood from the ventricle via inflow and outflow cannulas to the ascending aorta or by providing continuous support from inside the ventricular cavity or aorta. Available LV assist devices include:

- extracorporeal (pulsatile and non-pulsatile)
- implantable (pulsatile and non-pulsatile) (Figure 8.7)
- total artificial heart.

The pumps are either hydraulic or electromagnetic, and based on either an axial or centrifugal design. Most of the available systems operate at either fixed rates or in an automatic mode; the latter ejects when the pump is 90% full or when it senses decreased filling (more physiological). The aortic valve rarely opens when the heart is being supported, so pump output is synonymous with cardiac output. The devices can deliver cardiac output of up to 10 L/minute. The pump rhythm is completely dissociated from ventricular rhythm. The newest

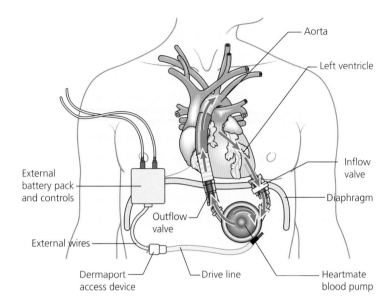

Figure 8.7 The Heartmate implantable left ventricle assist device (Thoratec Corporation, Pleasanton, CA, USA).

LV assist devices use a textured biological surface that does not require long-term anticoagulation.

The effect of LV assist devices on LV function has been extensively studied. At the cellular level the mechanical unloading attenuates myocardial histological abnormalities, improves the efficiency of mitochondria and decreases the extent of myocyte apoptosis.

Dramatic decreases in plasma renin, angiotensin II, epinephrine, norepinephrine, vasopressin and atrial natriuretic peptide have been observed, with inflammatory markers such as tumor necrosis factor (TNF), interleukin (IL)-6 and IL-8 beneficially affected by chronic support. At the organ level, there is reversal of LV remodeling with reduction in LV size, improvement in LVEF and regression of myocyte hypertrophy, and better hemodynamics, exercise tolerance and functional state.

Complications are frequent and potentially life-threatening. They differ according to the time of implantation (Table 8.4).

Pre-existing mitral stenosis or aortic regurgitation may require correction before implantation. Patients with inoperable coronary artery disease (CAD) sometimes continue to have angina.

TABLE 8.4

Complications associated with left ventricle assist devices

In early postoperative period	In late postoperative period
• Bleeding (30%)	• Infection (25%)
• Right-sided heart failure (10%)	• Thromboembolism
• Air embolism	• Failure of the device

The REMATCH trial compared the long-term effect of LV assist devices with medical therapy. The results supported the use of the devices for patients with advanced HF, but at the cost of device-related complications, including:

• 35% failure rate at 2 years (none after 1 year)
• 28% device infection rate after 3 months
• 42% bleeding rate after 6 months.

Median number of days spent both in and out of the hospital were higher in the device group.

Patient selection. There are three groups of patients who should be considered for LV assist devices.

• Patients who are not expected to recover adequate cardiac function and who require mechanical support as a bridge to transplantation.

• Patients who require ventricular assistance to allow the heart to rest and recover its function in preparation for explantation (bridge to recovery).

• Patients who require permanent LV support and are not eligible for cardiac transplantation (destination therapy).

Destination therapy enables long-term myocardial replacement therapy and in some cases, the patient's hemodynamic profile may improve to such an extent that heart replacement therapy could be reconsidered.

Extracorporeal membrane oxygenation (ECMO) has been a major step forward in the management of patients with acute severe pulmonary and cardiac failure. ECMO is a modified heart–lung machine that can support life for days or weeks, thereby allowing adequate time for treatment (including a bridge to implantation of an LV assist device, a total artificial heart [TAH] or cardiac transplantation) or myocardial recovery. There is already evidence of the positive impact of ECMO on outcomes in patients with refractory cardiogenic shock after surgery and following acute MI.

The total artificial heart is a mechanical device, made of plastic and metal, which replaces the heart's function. Although it is currently used as a bridge to transplantation, work continues to make it ready for potential destination therapy. A synthetic fully functional mechanical heart is one of the holy grails of medicine. While transplant recipients outnumber organ donors there will be a drive to develop this technology.

The first mechanical heart was used as a bridge to transplant in 1969. Since then, a number of versions of the device have been made. Studies show that up to 80% of patients survive to transplant. Newer prototypes using electronic sensors and 'biomaterials' such as chemically treated animal tissues are in the advanced stages of development and it is projected that in the long term totally implantable hearts will be available within the next 2–3 years.

Currently in use, the Food and Drug Administration (FDA)-approved SynCardia TAH is a biventricular, pneumatic pulsatile blood pump that completely replaces the patient's native ventricles. It is lined with polyurethane and has a pneumatically driven diaphragm (Figure 8.8).

The device is used as a bridge to transplantation in patients for whom LV assist and CRT devices are contraindicated, including those with aortic regurgitation, cardiac arrhythmias, a left ventricular thrombus, an aortic prosthesis, an acquired ventricular septal defect, or irreversible biventricular failure requiring high pump outputs. The device is powered by a large console that limits the patient's movement. Portable drivers that will enable patients to return home are in the testing phase.

Complications. As with all mechanical devices the two major complications are thromboembolism and infection. Although infection is common (up to 20% are device related), it is treatable and does not necessarily mandate device removal. Pulmonary infection is also common (up to 20%), as are neurological events (15%). Despite these complications, overall success has been increasing and these devices are becoming increasingly acceptable.

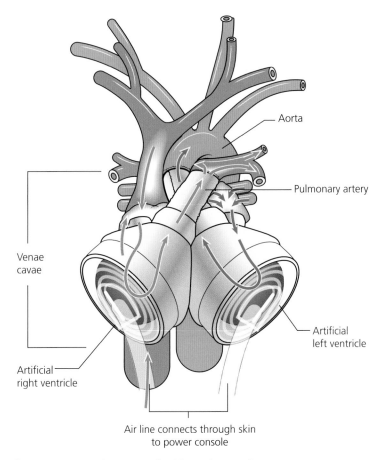

Aorta

Pulmonary artery

Venae cavae

Artificial left ventricle

Artificial right ventricle

Air line connects through skin to power console

Figure 8.8 SynCardia total artificial heart (SynCardia Systems Inc., Tucson, AZ, USA), a pulsatile blood pump that completely replaces the patient's right and left ventricles.

Cardiac support device. The CorCap cardiac support device is a latex-free polyester mesh jacket designed to be wrapped around the heart ventricles (Figure 8.9). It is used in patients with a severely dilated heart and symptoms of HF despite optimal treatment.

Although developed over 10 years ago it is not yet widely accepted, but has shown some promise. It promotes reverse remodeling of the left ventricle, reduces LV end systolic volumes, increases ejection fraction and improves quality of life. It is used as complementary therapy for particularly complex patients but requires further study to identify who benefits most.   113

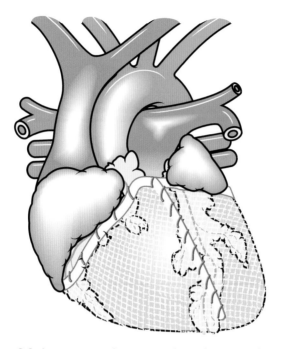

Figure 8.9 The CorCap cardiac support device (Acorn Cardiovascular, Inc., St Paul, MN, USA).

Cardiac transplantation outcomes have been steadily improving over the last 30 years. Currently, over 85% of patients will survive 12 months and 50% of transplant recipients are still alive at 10 years. Although highly successful, the major limitation is the availability of donor hearts. In the USA there are approximately 2500 transplants per year, 3500 worldwide, against an estimated 800 000 eligible people with end-stage HF. This mismatch in demand has spurred the development of other approaches to support a failing heart (see above).

Patient selection. Patients with severe HF who may benefit from transplantation (Table 8.5) should be referred to a heart transplant center for assessment of the severity of the disease process, to ensure that all other therapeutic options have been exhausted and to evaluate potential hazards or contraindications to the treatment. Patients who are considered for transplantation have to undergo a battery of tests.

Age is one of the most controversial exclusion criteria for transplantation (Table 8.6). The upper age limit for recipients is determined by the patient's physiological rather than chronological age, as older patients have a greater probability of occult systemic disease that may complicate their postoperative course and limit their survival.

TABLE 8.5

Indications for heart transplantation

- NYHA class III or IV heart failure refractory to optimized medical and surgical therapy as evidenced by:
  - peak oxygen consumption (VO_2max) < 14 mL/kg/min during cardiopulmonary exercise testing
- Refractory angina despite maximum therapy
- Life-threatening arrhythmias despite maximum therapy

TABLE 8.6

Exclusion criteria for heart transplantation

- Age > 70 years
- TPG > 15 mmHg or PVR > 6 Woods units if not reversible on vasodilator challenge
- Morbid obesity BMI ≥ 35, or cachexia BMI < 20
- Current alcohol, smoking or drug abuse
- Active malignancy
- Active systemic infection or peptic ulcer disease
- Uncontrolled hyperlipidemia
- Personality/behavioral disorder likely to affect treatment adherence
- Severe peripheral and cerebrovascular disease
- Severe osteoporosis
- Other medical condition likely to cause death within 5 years
- Diabetes mellitus with end-organ damage.
- Irreversible secondary organ disease (unless combined treatment is considered)

BMI, body mass index (kg/m^2); PVR, pulmonary vascular resistance; TPG, transpulmonary gradient.

Eligible patients are placed on the waiting lists. Those who are hemodynamically unstable are referred for mechanical support. Interestingly, improved preoperative care has meant that the death rate for patients awaiting cardiac transplantation has declined considerably.

The criteria for matching potential recipients with the appropriate donor are based primarily on ABO blood group compatibility and patient size (donor weight should be within 30% of the recipient). The panel of reactive antibodies (PRA) representing the major histocompatibility antigens is used to screen the recipient for antibodies that may mediate hyperacute rejection. If the PRA is greater than 15%, suggesting recipient presensitization, a prospective negative cross match between the recipient and donor sera is mandatory before transplantation.

After surgery, patients are placed on an intensive immunosuppressive regimen, including a calcineurin inhibitor (ciclosporin or tacrolimus), an antimetabolite (mycophenolate mofetil or azathioprine) and a corticosteroid. Prophylactic therapy against pneumocystis and cytomegalovirus (CMV)/toxoplasmosis infections is also given if the patient has been exposed previously. Transplantation is a major psychological trauma, and family and social support are key to a successful outcome. A life-long commitment to therapy and follow-up is required.

The commonest causes of morbidity and mortality after transplantation are listed in Table 8.7. Significant morbidity is also attributed to other

TABLE 8.7

Commonest causes of morbidity and mortality after heart transplantation

Within 30 days of transplant	After 1 year
• Rejection	• Coronary artery vasculopathy (in 50% at 5 years)
• Primary graft failure	
• Infection (mainly bacterial)	• Infection (mainly cytomegalovirus and fungal)
Within 1 year of transplant	• Malignancy (mainly skin and lymphomas)
• Infection	
• Rejection	
• Graft failure	

conditions resulting from the use of immunosuppressive therapy (mainly calcineurin inhibitors and steroids). These include arterial hypertension (~90% of recipients), diabetes mellitus (~30%), renal dysfunction (~30%) and hyperlipidemia (~85%).

Key points – non-pharmacological management

- Patients with poor left ventricular systolic function (ejection fraction < 35%), who are symptomatic on adequate treatment, with broad QRS complexes (> 120 ms) and left bundle branch block should be referred for cardiac resynchronization therapy.
- With evolving technology, the complication rate of left ventricle assist devices and total artificial hearts will decline and their use will significantly increase as a bridge to transplantation and as destination therapy.
- Assuming that the candidate pool (patients with end-stage HF) continues to grow, the burden on healthcare systems worldwide could become significant.
- Cardiac transplantation remains a viable option in selected individuals with end-stage HF despite the shortage of donor organs; steady improvement in survival after cardiac transplantation has been observed.

Key references

Jones RH, Velazquez EJ, Michler RE et al. Coronary bypass surgery with or without surgical ventricular reconstruction. *N Engl J Med* 2009;360:1705–17.

Moss AJ, Hall WJ, Cannom DS et al. Cardiac resynchronization therapy for the prevention of heart-failure events. *N Engl J Med* 2009;361:1329–38.

Rose EA, Gelijns AC, Moskowitz AJ et al. Long-term use of a left ventricular assist device for end-stage heart failure. *New Engl J Med* 2001;345:1435–43.

Solomon SD, Foster E, Bourgoun M et al. Effect of cardiac resynchronization therapy on reverse remodeling and relation to outcome: multicenter automatic defibrillator implantation trial: cardiac resynchronization therapy. *Circulation* 2010;122:985–92.

Diagnosis of heart failure (HF) carries a poor prognosis, often comparable with that of cancer (see Figure 1.3, page 13). The annual mortality for mild to moderate HF (NYHA class II or III) is 24–28%, and increases to 50% in patients with severe NYHA class IV symptoms. Hospital admission with acute HF is a strong and independent predictor of worse prognosis, and is associated with 2–4% in-hospital and 5–15% 90-day mortality. Between 30% and 50% of patients with acute HF are readmitted within 6 months, although 50% of these readmissions are due to comorbidities, often associated with advanced age, rather than existing HF.

Prognosis of HF in individual patients is challenging as a number of independent variables must be considered, including symptoms, severity, etiology and type of HF. The fact that sudden death can occur at any stage of the disease makes the prognostic process even less predictable. In general, patients with NYHA class IV symptoms, and HF caused by infiltrative heart disease, HIV infection or anthracycline toxicity, with systolic left ventricular (LV) or biventricular dysfunction, have the worse prognosis.

Outcomes are poor when the intensity of HF treatment is low and the patient does not adhere to the medications prescribed. Comorbidities (e.g. renal disease, diabetes mellitus), advanced age, male sex and ethnicity all contribute to worse outcomes.

Markers of poor prognosis

Several clinical and laboratory markers of poor prognosis have been validated (Table 9.1). Other identified factors of reduced survival in patients with HF include attenuated response to diuretics, low peak oxygen consumption (VO_2max) or short distance in the 6-Minute Walk Test (6MWT), a large burden of ventricular ectopy and complex ventricular arrhythmia, significant pulmonary hypertension, new-onset atrial fibrillation and specific echocardiographic features (significant LV dyssynchrony, evidence of ongoing remodeling and a marked increase in left atrial volume).

TABLE 9.1

Clinical and laboratory markers of poor prognosis*

Cardiac function

- LVEF < 20% (mortality doubles when LVEF drops from 35% to 17%)
- Abnormal RV systolic function

Hospitalization for heart failure

- Almost threefold increase in risk of death within 12 months after discharge
- Highest risk within 1 month of discharge

Hypotension

- Low mean arterial blood pressure (a 10-mmHg decrease is associated with an 11% increase in risk)

Low eGFR and serum sodium level

- Impaired renal function (e.g. patients with cardiorenal syndrome and hyponatremia)

Conduction disease

- Marked prolongation of QRS (> 150 ms) on surface ECG with evidence of LBBB morphology

Clinical findings

- S3 gallop (a third heart sound)
- Persistently elevated jugular venous pressure
- Elevated resting heart rate
- Weight loss

Neurohormones

- Chronically elevated plasma levels of norepinephrine (noradrenaline), epinephrine (adrenaline) and aldosterone
- High plasma renin activity
- Elevated BNP level
- Elevated troponin levels

(CONTINUED)

TABLE 9.1 (CONTINUED)

Autonomic dysfunction

- Reduced heart rate variability
- Poor baroreflex sensitivity
- Increased central and peripheral chemoreflex activation
- Activation of skeletal muscle ergoreceptors

Others

- Depression
- Hypoalbuminemia
- Hyperuricemia
- Hypocholesterolemia

*Reduced survival or higher mortality.
BNP, type B natriuretic peptide; eGFR, estimated glomerular filtration rate; LBBB, left bundle branch block; LVEF, left ventricular ejection fraction; RV, right ventricular.

Reversible factors

Initial assessment in patients with HF should include a review of the prognosis but, importantly, a search for reversible factors contributing to disease progression (Table 9.2). If any of these problems are identified, prompt and comprehensive treatment should improve HF symptoms, in many cases arrest the progression of the disease and improve the prognosis.

Palliative care in end-stage heart failure

Palliative care improves the quality of life of patients and their families facing the problems associated with life-threatening illness. This is accomplished by the prevention and relief of symptoms, including early identification, assessment and treatment of pain and other physical, psychosocial and spiritual problems (Table 9.3).

The quality of life of patients with advanced HF refractory to optimal pharmacological and non-pharmacological strategies can be very poor and comparable with that of patients with terminal malignancies, with a case–fatality rate of 75% over 5 years overall.

In general, an illness trajectory for HF can provide a broad estimate of timeframe and help to predict patterns of need and interaction with health and social services (Figure 9.1).

TABLE 9.2

Reversible factors that contribute to disease progression

- Non-adherence to treatment
- Cardiac arrhythmia
- Myocardial ischemia
- Arterial hypertension
- Cardiac dyssynchrony
- Thyroid disease
- Alcohol abuse

TABLE 9.3

The principles of palliative care

- Provides relief from pain and other distressing symptoms
- Affirms life and regards dying as a normal process
- Intends neither to hasten nor postpone death
- Integrates the psychological and spiritual aspects of patient care
- Offers a support system to help patients live as actively as possible until death
- Offers a support system to help the family cope during the patient's illness and in their own bereavement
- Uses a team approach to address the needs of patients and their families,
- Enhances quality of life and positively influences the course of illness
- Is applicable early in the course of illness, in conjunction with other therapies that are intended to prolong life and includes those investigations needed to better understand and manage distressing clinical complications.

Adapted from the WHO 2004 definition of palliative care; available at www.who.int/cancer/palliative/en, last accessed 12 July 2012.

In practical terms advanced HF can be divided into three distinct stages:

- chronic disease management
- palliative and supportive care
- terminal care.

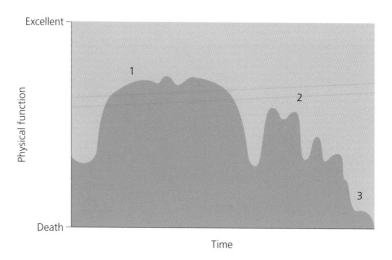

Figure 9.1 Illness trajectory, showing the distinct stages of clinical heart failure. (1) The overall stable functional status of chronic disease management. (2) Palliative and supportive care, during which clinical exacerbation leads to progressive deterioration in physical functioning. (3) Terminal care. Adapted from Goodlin SJ. 2009.

Chronic disease management strategies include education, monitoring, prevention and effective therapy (see earlier chapters). They are used to prolong life, prevent HF hospitalization and provide symptomatic relief. Intervention should be delivered using the protocols of locally available HF management programs. Patients and their families (carers) should be fully informed about the nature of the disease including treatment and prognosis, with regular monitoring and appropriate review.

Palliative and supportive care may begin following readmission to hospital with HF. A careful review of the patient's symptoms and all the available treatment options should be performed by the specialist in consultation with the patient's family practitioner and a palliative care specialist, using robust clinical identifiers of poor prognosis (Table 9.4).

If the patient assessment indicates the need for palliative care, management should shift to symptom control (Table 9.5). Patients and their families or carers may require assistance in negotiating the change in goals of care from prolongation of life to improvement of quality of life by

TABLE 9.4

Identifiers of patients with advanced heart failure and poor prognosis

- Patient with consistent NYHA class IV HF
  - unable to undertake physical activity without discomfort
  - symptoms of chronic HF present at rest
  - severe chronic HF

and

- Not suitable for any further procedures, such as:
  - revascularization with coronary bypass surgery
  - coronary angioplasty
  - valve surgery
  - cardiac resynchronization therapy (biventricular pacing [BiV-P])
  - heart transplantation

plus, at least one of:

- increasing HF symptoms despite maximum tolerated HF therapy, including diuretics, ACE inhibitors and beta-blockers, as indicated
- worsening or irreversible end-organ damage (including cardiac cachexia)
- repeated hospital readmissions with deteriorating HF, ventricular arrhythmias or cardiac arrest

ACE, angiotensin-converting enzyme; HF, heart failure; NYHA, New York Heart Association.

maximizing comfort and dignity. Time should be set aside to discuss the prognosis, course of the illness and palliative-care strategies in detail with the patient and carer. A program of care individualized to the needs of the patient and their family is extremely important. Palliative-care strategies should build on, rather than replace, multidisciplinary programs of care that optimize advanced HF management. Properly applied, they can cut the overall cost of care by reducing the amount of time patients spend in acute-care settings.

TABLE 9.5

Management of symptoms in the palliative-care phase of advanced heart failure

Dyspnea

- Assess all causes and exclude reversible reasons
- Involve physiotherapist in review of breathing techniques
- Offer psychological support
- Consider anxiety therapy
- Include relaxation techniques
- Provide fans and recliner beds
- Use of home oxygen
- Introduce opioids with oral morphine initially, 2–3 mg, and titrate according to response; initial use when required, may change to long-acting (always use prophylactic laxatives)
- Set up nebulizers – with saline and bronchodilators
- Consider glyceryl trinitrate and sublingual lorazepam

Nausea and vomiting

- Exclude drug(s) as a cause
- If constant, start haloperidol, 1–3 mg orally, olanzapine or levomepromazine
- If meal-related, introduce metoclopramide, 10 mg tds
- Review delivery methods; administer subcutaneously if symptoms persistent or vomiting

Pain

- Perform full assessment of cause
- Introduce an oral opioid with slow dose titration (use prophylactic laxatives)
- Exclude and/or treat gout
- Avoid NSAIDs

(CONTINUED)

TABLE 9.5 (CONTINUED)

Mood disorder/anxiety/insomnia

- Consider antidepressants (sertraline, citalopram, mirtazapine) but avoid tricyclics
- Use night sedation with lorazepam or temazepam (if indicated)
- Start anxiolytics – lorazepam or diazepam if anxiety is a large component
- Explore underlying psychosocial and spiritual issues

Peripheral edema

- Continue primary therapy with diuretics unless resistant to therapy
- Use emollients for the involved skin
- Consider bandaging with gradual pressure in massive edema
- Involve OT techniques (appropriate posture and rest) and massage
- Provide scrotal supports (if indicated)

NSAID, non-steroidal anti-inflammatory drug. OT, occupational therapy; tds, three times daily.

Clear communication with community-care providers and family members should always precede any changes in directions or content of care provided by the treating team. An advance care plan is often documented and the ways of managing future clinical deterioration discussed with the patient. Carers should be included in the management plans.

Advanced health directive. Recognizing that the outcomes of resuscitation in patients with advanced HF are dismal, individuals should be empowered to express their treatment preferences even when unable to speak for themselves. The existence and process of obtaining such a legal document should be discussed with the patient and their carers early in the course of advanced HF.

Medication withdrawal. As the patient's condition deteriorates, the healthcare team should discuss any changes to the goals of medical therapy with the patient and family. This inevitably will include review of the current medical therapy and termination of non-essential drugs. The list includes but is not limited to statins, acetylsalicylic acid (ASA;

aspirin) and warfarin, vasodilators and beta-blockers (especially in patients with low blood pressure), aldosterone antagonists, anti-anginals and other therapies for comorbidities.

Device deactivation. Automatic implantable cardiac defibrillators (ICDs) have become a common therapeutic option in suitable patients with severe HF. They can help prevent sudden cardiac death, but in advanced HF they can become a potential cause of distress when incessant ventricular rhythms develop. In these circumstances, the patient's quality of life should be paramount, and in many instances deactivation of the device may need to be discussed. To prepare patients and their families for such meetings, many physicians explore these issues at the time of implantation and continue to monitor the patient's status during follow-up visits. If progression to advanced HF becomes clear it is suggested that discussion regarding deactivation of the ICD function should take place. In many instances the 'not-for-resuscitation' status and arrangements for terminal care are also reviewed at this time (see below).

Terminal care continues as the patient presents with intractable HF, with resting symptoms, poor appetite, weight loss, slow mental activity and low blood pressure with end-organ failure (e.g. kidney failure). Therapy for symptom control should continue. The patient's resuscitation status should be reviewed with the patient and carer, and documented (see page 125). Carers will require increased practical and emotional support, followed by bereavement support.

Key points – prognosis

- Heart failure (HF) has a poor prognosis with an annual mortality of 25–50% depending on severity of symptoms and left ventricular (LV) systolic dysfunction.
- Poor prognostic signs include impaired renal function, marked prolongation of QRS, hypotension and hyponatremia.
- The search for reversible factors is always indicated.
- The model of palliative care for advanced HF needs to be very flexible, individualized to the needs of the patient and their family.
- Good communication skills are the key to effective palliative care delivery.
- Primary care, cardiology and palliative care teams should work in collaboration to deliver an effective phase-specific treatment in advanced HF.
- End-of-life planning and decision making are essential and should be discussed early in the process.

Key references

Goodlin SJ. Palliative care in congestive heart failure. *J Am Coll Cardiol* 2009;54:386–96.

Jaarsma T, Beattie JM, Ryder M et al. Palliative care in heart failure: a position statement from the palliative care workshop of the Heart Failure Association of the European Society of Cardiology. *Eur J Heart Fail* 2009;11:433–43.

Piepoli M. Diagnostic and prognostic indicators in chronic HF. [Editorial] *Eur Heart J* 1999;20:1367–9.

This chapter presents the results of recent studies, and reviews the design of new trials in patients with systolic and diastolic heart failure (HF), both chronic and acute.

New drugs for systolic heart failure

Direct renin inhibitors. The renin–angiotensin–aldosterone system becomes pathologically activated in patients with HF (see Chapter 2) and several drugs have been developed to block its action (angiotensin-converting enzyme [ACE] inhibitors, aldosterone antagonists). However, an escape mechanism via alternative enzyme pathways can lead to ongoing system activity. The ATMOSPHERE trial has been designed to evaluate the effects of aliskiren (direct renin inhibitor) and enalapril (ACE inhibitor) monotherapies and aliskiren/enalapril combination therapy on cardiovascular death and HF hospitalization in patients with chronic systolic HF (NYHA class II–IV) and elevated plasma levels of BNP (type B natriuretic peptide).

The primary endpoints of this ongoing non-inferiority study are times to first occurrence of cardiovascular death or HF hospitalization.

Xanthine oxidase inhibition. Oxidative stress may contribute to ventricular and vascular remodeling and disease progression in patients with HF. Xanthine oxidase is a potential source of oxidative stress in HF, and may be an important target for therapy. Allopurinol, a xanthine oxidase inhibitor that reduces serum uric acid levels, may be useful in the treatment of patients with systolic HF, left ventricular ejection fraction (LVEF) less than 40%, NYHA class II–IV and elevated serum uric acid levels.

The EXACT study has a composite clinical endpoint that includes symptoms and death, hospitalization and medication change for worsening HF.

New drugs for heart failure with preserved ejection fraction

Aldosterone antagonist. TOPCAT is a multicenter international randomized double-blind placebo-controlled trial of the aldosterone antagonist spironolactone in patients with HF and LVEF above 45%. The primary endpoint is a composite of cardiovascular mortality, aborted cardiac arrest or hospitalization for the management of HF. Secondary endpoints include all-cause mortality, new-onset diabetes mellitus or atrial fibrillation and quality of life.

Phosphodiesterase-5 inhibitor. RELAX is a double-blind placebo-controlled clinical trial of chronic phosphodiesterase (PDE)-5 inhibition with sildenafil (20 mg three times daily for 12 weeks followed by 60 mg three times daily for 12 weeks) in patients with HF and preserved LVEF. The primary endpoint is the change in exercise capacity as assessed by peak oxygen consumption (VO_2max) after 24 weeks of treatment with the PDE-5 inhibitor or placebo.

Device trials

Cardiac resynchronization therapy in heart failure and narrow QRS. EchoCRT is a large-scale prospective randomized clinical outcome trial to assess cardiac resynchronization therapy (CRT) in patients with symptomatic HF, LVEF less than 35%, narrow QRS (< 130 ms) and echocardiography evidence of cardiac dyssynchrony. Primary endpoints include a combination of cardiovascular death and HF readmission.

Hemodynamic monitoring. There is increased interest in hemodynamic monitoring to predict acute HF decompensation. Direct or indirect measurement of intracardiac pressures and long-term pulmonary pressure monitoring is under investigation.

Total artificial heart. The SynCardia total artificial heart (TAH) is a Food and Drug Administration (FDA)-approved bridge-to-transplantation device for patients with severe biventricular HF (see pages 112–13). A new trial is currently evaluating the SynCardia Freedom Driver, which will enable TAH patients to return home while awaiting a suitable cardiac donor.

Surgery – new indications and techniques

Surgical revascularization in ischemic cardiomyopathy. The STICH Coronary Artery Bypass Graft (CABG) study compared the effects of surgical revascularization and medical therapy in patients with severe HF

129

(LVEF < 35%), with about 5 years of follow up. The surgical group had a lower rate of death from cardiovascular causes, and a lower composite endpoint of death and cardiovascular rehospitalization.

Mitral valve intervention in severe mitral valve regurgitation. MitraClip is a new technology exploiting the surgical technique of the Alfieri stitch (the fusion of anterior and posterior mitral valve leaflets). The clip is delivered percutaneously. EVEREST was the first randomized trial to compare the outcome of MitraClip and surgery in patients with severe regurgitation. The primary outcome (freedom from death, surgery and grade 3+/4+ regurgitation) was better in the surgical group, but the safety endpoint (need for blood transfusions) was reduced in the MitraClip group.

New therapies in acute decompensated heart failure

Calcium sensitizers. Levosimendan has been reported to enhance cardiac performance by calcium sensitization (of structural protein troponin C) combined with vasodilatation via ATP-dependent potassium channels. The data suggest symptomatic improvement in the short term in subjects with acute decompensated HF but no impact on mortality over placebo, and similar mortality rates to dobutamine.

Direct myosin activators. Omecamtiv mecarbil has been found to increase LV contractility and cardiac output without significant change in intracellular calcium currents, myocardial oxygen uptake or coronary blood flow. ATOMIC AHF is a prospective double-blind placebo-controlled trial in patients with severe HF, LVEF below 40% and acute admission requiring intravenous diuretic therapy. The primary endpoint is level of dyspnea at 48 hours after drug infusion.

Ultrafiltration in cardiorenal syndrome. The CARRESS study is a randomized controlled trial of ultrafiltration versus pharmacological care in patients with acute decompensated HF and cardiorenal syndrome (defined as an increase in serum creatinine ≥ 0.3 mg/dL from baseline). The primary endpoint is change in serum creatinine and weight together ('bivariate' endpoint) at days 1, 2, 3, 4 and 7.

Renal optimization strategies in cardiorenal syndrome. ROSE is a randomized double-blind placebo-controlled multicenter clinical trial of patients with signs and symptoms consistent with acute decompensated HF within 24 hours of hospital admission. There are three treatment regimens:

- optimal diuretic dosing and placebo
- optimal diuretic dosing and low-dose dopamine
- optimal diuretic dosing and low-dose nesiritide.

Primary endpoints include the change in level of serum cystatin C and cumulative urinary volume 72 hours from randomization.

Istaroxime has lusitropic and inotropic actions via sodium/potassium ATP pump inhibition and specific receptor (SERCA-2) stimulation. Preliminary data in patients with acute decompensated HF with LVEF below 35% demonstrated a significant decrease in pulmonary wedge pressure, an increase in blood pressure and cardiac index, and a decrease in heart rate. An increase in systolic and decrease in diastolic elastance led to improved compliance.

New oral anticoagulants

Dabigatran is an oral reversible direct thrombin inhibitor. In the RELY study, dabigatran, 150 mg twice daily, was superior to warfarin (1.11%/year versus 1.69%/year) in preventing systemic embolism in patients with non-valvular atrial fibrillation, about 30% of whom had either LVEF below 40% or symptomatic HF. A lower dose of 110 mg twice daily was non-inferior to warfarin in preventing systemic embolism (1.53%/year versus 1.69%/year), but caused fewer bleeding complications.

Close monitoring has been recommended in patients over 75 years of age, and in patients with low bodyweight and renal dysfunction (as an excess in bleeding episodes has been reported). No antidote currently exists.

Rivaroxaban is a reversible factor Xa inhibitor in once-daily oral formulation. The ROCKET AF study confirmed non-inferiority of rivaroxaban, 20 mg, to warfarin (2.12%/year versus 2.42%/year) in preventing systemic embolism in patients with non-valvular atrial fibrillation. About 60% of patients in this study had HF.

131

Stem cell therapy

Stem cell therapy remains a promising treatment for patients with LV dysfunction after myocardial infarction (MI). Intracoronary or intramyocardial injections of skeletal myoblasts or bone-marrow-derived mononuclear cells have led to a modest improvement in cardiac performance in some studies, but the clinical effect of such therapies has not yet been proven. The therapy appears to be well tolerated in patients after recent MI, but a proarrhythmic effect of cell therapy has been observed in patients with chronic HF.

Recently, it has been demonstrated that the delivered cells may secrete substances that exert a protective effect on the ischemic myocardium. Intensive work in this and other areas (including the type of cell used, and the method and time of delivery) continues, with randomized trials recruiting in Europe and the USA. However, stem cell therapy is not yet ready to become a mainstay of clinical practice.

Key points – clinical trials and developments

- Promising trials of new compounds for the management of acute and chronic systolic and diastolic heart failure (HF) are due for completion in 2013.
- An important study assessing cardiac resynchronization therapy in HF with narrow QRS is ongoing.
- The use of ultrafiltration and low-dose dopamine support in cardiorenal syndrome awaits validation.
- Intensive research in the areas of cell therapy and total artificial heart continues.

Useful resources

UK
British Cardiovascular Society
+44 (0)20 7383 3887
enquiries@bcs.com
www.bcs.com

British Heart Foundation
Tel: +44 (0)20 7554 0000
www.bhf.org.uk

British Society for Heart Failure
Tel: +44 (0)1865 391836
info@bsh.org.uk
www.bsh.org.uk

Primary Care Cardiovascular
Society
Tel: +44 (0)20 8994 8775
office@pccs.org.uk
www.pccs.org.uk

USA
American College of Cardiology
Tel: +1 202 375 6000
resource@acc.org
www.cardiosource.org

American Heart Association
Toll-free: 1 800 242 8721
www.heart.org
www.hearthub.org

Heart Failure Society of America
Tel: +1 651 642 1633
info@hfsa.org
www.hfsa.org

International
Canadian Cardiovascular Society
Toll-free: 1 877 569 3407
Tel: +1 613 569 3407
info@ccs.ca
www.ccs.ca

Cardiac Society of Australia and
New Zealand
Tel: +61 2 9256 5452
info@csanz.edu.au
www.csanz.edu.au

European Society of Cardiology
Tel: +33 4 92 94 76 00
www.escardio.org
www.heartfailurematters.org

Heart Foundation (Australia)
Toll-free: 1300 36 27 87
www.heartfoundation.org.au

Further reading

Driving regulations

American Medical Association. *Physician's Guide to Assessing and Counseling Older Drivers*, 2nd edn, 2010. Available from www.ama-assn.org/ama1/pub/upload/mm/433/older-drivers-guide.pdf, last accessed 23 July 2012.

Austroads. *Assessing Fitness to Drive* (Australia). www.austroads.com.au/assessing-fitness-to-drive, last accessed 23 July 2012.

Driver and Vehicle Licensing Agency (UK). Guidance available at www.dft.gov.uk/dvla/medical/medical_professionals.aspx, last accessed 23 July 2012.

Other guidelines

Dickstein K, Cohen-Solal A, Filippatos G et al. ESC guidelines for the diagnosis and treatment of acute and chronic heart failure 2008: the Task Force for the diagnosis and treatment of acute and chronic heart failure 2008 of the European Society of Cardiology. Developed in collaboration with the Heart Failure Association of the ESC (HFA) and endorsed by the European Society of Intensive Care Medicine (ESICM). *Eur J Heart Fail* 2008;10:933–89.

Dickstein K, Vardas PE, Auricchio A et al. 2010 Focused Update of ESC Guidelines on device therapy in heart failure: an update of the 2008 ESC Guidelines for the diagnosis and treatment of acute and chronic heart failure and the 2007 ESC guidelines for cardiac and resynchronization therapy. Developed with the special contribution of the Heart Failure Association and the European Heart Rhythm Association. *Eur Heart J* 2010;31:2677–87.

Heart Failure Society of America, Lindenfeld J, Albert NM et al. HFSA 2010 Comprehensive Heart Failure Practice Guideline. *J Card Fail* 2010;16:e1–194.

Hunt SA, Abraham WT, Chin MH et al. 2009 Focused update incorporated into the ACC/AHA 2005 Guidelines for the Diagnosis and Management of Heart Failure in Adults: a report of the American College of Cardiology Foundation/American Heart Association Task Force on Practice Guidelines: developed in collaboration with the International Society for Heart and Lung Transplantation. *Circulation* 2009;119:e391–479.

National Heart Foundation of Australia and the Cardiac Society of Australia and New Zealand (Chronic Heart Failure Guidelines Expert Writing Panel). *Guidelines for the prevention, detection and management of chronic heart failure in Australia*. Updated October 2011. Available from www.heartfoundation.org.au/SiteCollectionDocuments/Chronic_Heart_Failure_Guidelines_2011.pdf, last accessed 23 July 2012.

Index

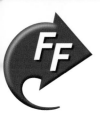
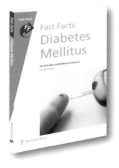
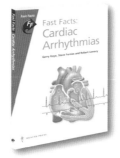
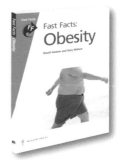
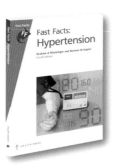
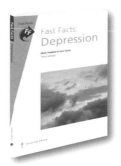
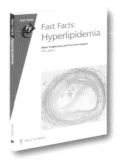
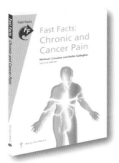
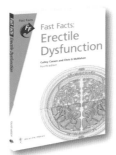
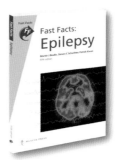

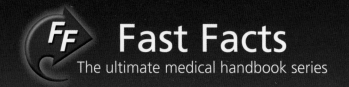

Our hope is that this Fast Facts *title helps you to improve your practice and, in turn, improves the health of your patients*

What will you do next?

Use this space to write some action points that have come from reading this book. And don't worry if you pass this on to a colleague, senior or junior; they are bound to find them interesting and may wish to add their own.

Action Point 1

Action Point 2

Action Point 3

If you have the time to share them with us, or you have suggestions of how to improve the next edition, we'd love to hear from you at **feedback@fastfacts.com**